The Potato Antioxidant:

ALPHA LIPOIC ACID

A Health Learning Handbook
By Beth M. Ley

BL Publications
Aliso Viejo, CA

BL Publications, Aliso Viejo, CA 92656
(714) 452-0371

Library of Congress Cataloging- In Publication Data
Ley, Beth M. 1964-
The potato antioxidant: alpha lipoic acid: a health learning handbook / by Beth M. Ley --1st edition.
    p.   cm.
    Includes bibliographical references and index.
    ISBN: 0-9642703-6-6
    1. Thiotic acid--physiological effect. 2. Thiotic acid-- health aspects. I. Title.
QP722.T54L48 1996
612' .01575--dc20   96-44738
                                 CIP

Printed in the United States of America

First edition, October 1996

The Potato Antioxidant: Alpha Lipoic Acid is not intended as medical advice. Its intention is solely informational and educational. It is wise to consult your doctor for any illness or medical condition.

Credits:
Typesetting and Cover Design: BL Publications
Editing: Kim DeLaura, Victoria Earhart, Sylvia Nelson

Technical assistance: Dr. Lester Packer, Mark Olsen
Additional thank-you's: Andrew Fischman, *NatureWorks* and, of course, my ever-patient husband, Randy.

TABLE OF CONTENTS

Introduction 5

Introduction to Free Radicals and Antioxidants 7

Free Radical Diseases 13

In Search of the Perfect Antioxidant 23

Cancer and α–Lipoic Acid 33

α–Lipoic Acid and Inflammatory Conditions 39
    Allergies, Asthma, Arthritis, etc.

Diabetes and α–Lipoic Acid 49

Neuroprotective Effects of α–Lipoic Acid 57

α–Lipoic Acid and the Eye 65
    Cataracts, Macular Degeneration, etc.

α–Lipoic Acid and HIV 75

α–Lipoic Acid and Heart Disease/LDL Cholesterol . .79

α–Lipoic Acid Protects Internal Organs. 83

α–Lipoic Acid as a Nutritional Supplement 89

Questions and Answers 91

Bibliography 97

Index 109

DEDICATION:

This book is dedicated to my grandparents, Pete and Esther Buttke, both in their 90's, living in Valley City, N.D.

Over a year ago, with the publication of *DHEA: Unlocking the Secrets to The Fountain of Youth*, my grandmother said to me, "*You really should write a book about taking care of the eyes.*"

A smoker for 50+ years, it was never revealed to her that cigarettes could rob her of her sight. Almost 25 years ago the battle began with cataracts, followed by surgery, glaucoma, surgery, complications and more surgery.

"*In life we may lose a lot of things, but the loss of one's sight is perhaps the worst.*"

Introduction

Health Learning Handbooks are designed to provide useful information about ways to improve one's health and well-being. Our intention is to help you learn about what the body needs in order to obtain and maintain good health.

Good health should not be thought of as the absence of disease. We should avoid negative disease-oriented thinking and concentrate on what we must do to remain healthy. Health is maintaining on a daily basis what is essential to the body. Disease is the result of attempting to live without what the body needs. We are responsible for our own health and should take control of it. If we are in control of our health, disease will not take control.

Our health depends on education.

Alpha Lipoic Acid (α-Lipoic Acid) is a vitamin-like antioxidant which is produced naturally in the body. We have known about its existence since the 1930's when it was discovered that a so-called "potato growth factor" was necessary for growth of certain bacteria. In 1957, the compound was extracted and formally identified as α-Lipoic Acid.

Through years of research, the unique metabolic antioxidant properties of α-Lipoic Acid have been clearly demonstrated and, while it is not yet a widely known substance, this is sure to change soon.

5

α–Lipoic Acid holds promise as a free radical protectant for our cells as it is the only antioxidant which is both fat and water soluble. α-Lipoic Acid is easily absorbed and transported across cell membranes. This capability offers us protection against free radical damage both inside and outside the cell. This is unlike many other antioxidants which provide only extracellular protection.

Cofactor for energy production: Under normal conditions, α-Lipoic Acid functions as a cofactor for a number of vital enzymes responsible for metabolism of our food to chemical energy (ATP). α-Lipoic Acid acts as a coenzyme at the active site of enzyme complexes.

Naturally found in foods we eat every day: Outside the body, α-Lipoic Acid is found in the leaves of plants containing mitochrondria and in non-photosynthetic plant tissues, such as potatoes, carrots, yams ans sweet potatoes. Red meat is also a very rich source of naturally-occurring α– Lipoic Acid.

Therapeutic applications*:* α-Lipoic Acid has been used throughout Europe to treat and prevent complications associated with **diabetes** including **neuropathy, macular degeneration and cataracts.**

An abundance of promising research has also shown the ability of α-Lipoic Acid to inhibit replication of HIV and other viruses, protect the liver and other organs, remove heavy metals, and also prevent damage from radiation.

In any situation in the body involving free radicals, including cancer, heart disease, and problems involving inflammation such as arthritis, asthma, allergies, etc., α-Lipoic Acid can be of great benefit. These situations are discussed in detail in this book.

Introduction to
Free Radicals and Antioxidants

Just 10 or 15 years ago, free radicals were little known to most of us. Researchers now tell us that free radical damage throughout the body is a major cause of aging and age-associated disease.

A free radical is an unstable, incomplete molecule. It is incomplete because it is missing an electron which exists in pairs in stable molecules. Free radicals are unstable because they "steal" an electron from another molecule, and thereby create another free radical and a chain reaction of events, which results in thousands of reactions.

Oxidation and Reduction (Redox)

Oxidation occurs when a molecule loses an electron. **Reduction** occurs when a molecule gains an electron. Reducing power refers to the ability of a compound to donate an electron - to reduce another compound. If a compound donates electrons easily, it has a high reducing power.

Every time molecules lose or gain an electron, the molecules are weakened and, ultimately, the whole structure, whether it is an enzyme, a protein, a cell membrane, tissues, or even organs, is damaged. Some areas of the body are more susceptible to damage than others.

Cell membrane damage can lead to numerous degenerative problems and accelerated aging. Free radicals are major factors in about 80 different diseases, including heart disease, cancer, diabetes, cataracts, macular degeneration, Alzheimer's, and inflammatory-related diseases, such as arthritis, lupus, asthma, etc.

Free Radicals Accelerate Aging

Aging also results from the loss of vital cells from free radical reactions. With each cell destroyed and without the ability to renew itself, we become one cell older. Free radicals can attack and damage cells from the inside or outside of the cell.

Free radicals age the body in at least five ways:

outside the cell

1. **Lipid peroxidation**. Free radicals damage fatty compounds circulating in the blood stream, causing damage and the release of more free radicals in a chain reaction.

outside the cell

2. **Membrane damage.** Free radicals destroy the integrity of cell membranes, interfering with the cell's ability to absorb nutrients and expel waste products. Without this ability, the cell dies.

inside and outside the cell

3. **Cross-linking.** When free radicals damage molecules, cells split off to repair the injury. The cells have to rejoin with others to reform and reshape themselves. This may cause cross linkage, a bond between large amino acid molecules which are normally separate from each other. Additional free radicals are also formed when waste fragments of these molecules break off. Most people are familiar with cross-linkages as a cause of wrinkles, but they also cause "aging" throughout the entire body. Free radicals cause proteins (i.e., collagen tissue) and/or genetic material (i.e., DNA) to fuse. Healthy DNA is necessary to replicate and renew the

8

body's cellular components. Altered DNA produces useless debris and sometimes cancerous cells.

inside the cell 4. **Lysosomal damage.** Free radicals destroy the membranes of lysosomes, enzyme-containing organelles found inside most cells. If the membrane sac that stores these enzymes is ruptured, the enzymes will kill the cell.

inside and outside the cell 5. Miscellaneous free radical reactions form residues called lipofuscin or age pigment. These residues accumulate with time and interfere with cell function and life processes.

Oxygen Free Radicals

One type of free radical in the body is toxic oxygen molecules, referred to as oxidants. Many oxidants are actually formed in the body naturally. While we think of oxygen as vital to existence, it is also responsible for the destruction and aging of all living things. Similar to the effect where iron is oxidized to rust, oxygen in its toxic state is able to oxidize molecules in our bodies. Compounds which prevent this process are called **antioxidants.**

Production of oxygen free radicals is a normal part of the body's mechanism. There are tens of thousands of free radicals formed in the body every second. However, they are not all harmful; some actually help us. The body's immune system uses free radicals to kill potentially infectious microbes and viruses. This activity is known as phagocytosis. This activity, however, at the same time creates even more free radicals (hydrogen peroxide and hydroxyl radicals) that may lead to severe tissue damage.

As long as the ratio of oxidants to antioxidants remains in balance, the negative effects of the free radicals can be controlled. When the balance becomes upset by

9

Antioxidant and Enzyme Cellular Protection

Inside and outside cellular membranes

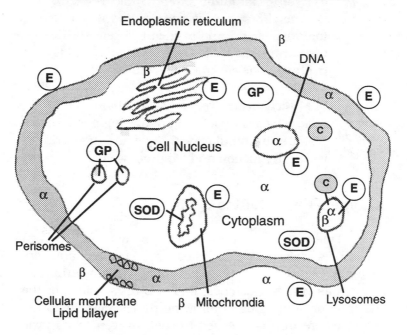

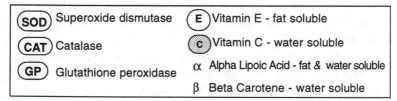

(SOD) Superoxide dismutase	(E) Vitamin E - fat soluble
(CAT) Catalase	(C) Vitamin C - water soluble
(GP) Glutathione peroxidase	α Alpha Lipoic Acid - fat & water soluble
	β Beta Carotene - water soluble

excessive exposure to internal or external factors or a combination of both, the antioxidants produced by the body simply cannot cope with the increased amount of free radicals.

Internal factors include chronic elevated glucose (as in diabetes) or chronic inflammation. Our daily exposure to environmental free radicals is a major contributor to production of free radicals in the body.

Oxygen free radicals are formed by molecular oxygen which is reduced in the body to water. The intermediate products formed during oxygen reduction are even more dangerous, including superoxide radicals, hydrogen peroxide, or the extremely damaging hydroxyl radical which reacts with anything it touches. Approximately 5 to 10% of the oxygen we breathe is converted to such radicals.

We are composed of molecules which make up proteins, membranes (consisting of readily oxidizable phospholipids), and polymers (made up of carbohydrates and nucleic acids). These and all other compounds and tissues in the body are susceptible to attack from reactive oxygen radicals.

Oxidants

O_2 - Superoxide radicals - We continuously form these as a part of cellular energy production and immune response, but they also come from irradiation, car exhaust, cigarette smoke and ozone. O_2 can be converted by iron or copper to the more toxic OH.

OH - Hydroxl radicals and Hydroperoxy radicals - the most aggressive and damaging species known.

NO - Nitrous oxide - reacts with oxygen to form the more damaging oxidant, nitrogen dioxide (NO_2).

O_3 - Ozone - an air pollutant.

O - Singlet Oxygen, like superoxide radicals, is produced in the body through various means.

Antioxidants

Antioxidants are a class of nutrients which possess the ability to destroy free radicals and thus prevent the diseases associated with free radical damage. Antioxidant

11

nutrients also help alleviate the symptoms and side-effects of many of these diseases. The following are the major antioxidant vitamins:

Vitamin E (α-tocopherol) is a major fat-soluble membrane antioxidant found in cells which fights off damage from peroxyl radicals.

Vitamin C (ascorbic acid) is effective against hydroxyl and superoxide radicals.

β-**carotene,** which is just one of about 50 different carotenoids, is effective against singlet oxygen. It is a "weak" antioxidant compared to Vitamins E and C. β-carotene is one of the few carotenoids which can convert to Vitamin A, a fat-soluble antioxidant. Vitamin A is ineffective against singlet oxygen.

The following increase your need for antioxidants:

1. Exercise.

2. Stress.

3. Exposure to pollutants, smog, poisons; i.g., tobacco smoke, alcohol, drugs and pesticides.

4. Illness, infection, inflammation, and many health problems: i.g., diabetes, arthritis, asthma.

5. Elevated blood lipids (especially LDL), elevated blood sugar.

6. Many stimulants and metabolic enhancers such as caffeine and diet pills.

7. Radiation (including UV light).

Some scientists believe that the reason humans live longer than chimpanzees, cats, dogs and other mammals is that we have a higher level of antioxidants within our cells. (Culter) The reason some people live longer than others is perhaps because they have higher levels of antioxidants within their cells protecting them from damage and disease.

Free Radical Diseases

The Mayo Clinic reports that approximately 43% of deaths in the United States are due to some form of cardiovascular disease, and 23% are caused by cancer. This is two of every three persons.

We now see the critical role which free radicals play in the development of both diseases. Low levels of antioxidants, which increase free radical activity, are clearly associated with an increased risk of these diseases. Therefore, the use of antioxidant supplements to scavenge free radicals can potentially decrease the risks of cancer, cardiovascular disease and many other degenerative health problems. (Barber)

We do not yet fully understand exactly how free radicals cause oxidative damage to cells and tissues. These radicals act on different structures, and the use of various antioxidants exert various favorable effects. Our genetics may make us sensitive to certain health problems such as heart disease or diabetes, but location of the free radical exposure or formation also plays a significant role in the type of damage which results. For example, UV exposure is damaging to the skin and the eyes, elevated LDL cholesterol molecules circulating in our veins are more susceptible to damage creating arterial plague to buildup. Smoking damages the throat and lungs, etc.

Free radicals attack three types of molecules:

1. Polyunsaturated fatty acids

Destroys cell membranes which are made up of these sensitive fatty acids.

Damages LDL and Lipoprotein(a) which are associated with heart disease.

2. DNA

Genetic material which is associated with cell abnormalities and cancer.

3. Proteins

Protein destruction as seen in cataract formation, kidney damage, and damage to hemoglobin cells and aging in general (collagen breakdown).

The physico-chemical properties of radicals and their electronic structure are precisely known. In the organism they are formed in side reactions of the respiratory chain. When the electron transfer is not optimally coordinated, electrons accumulate at certain stages of the reaction, with a consequent oxidation and peroxidation of the inner mitochondrial membrane.

The main targets for free radical attack are the vulnerable lipid-composed membranes of cells and their inner structures: the mitochondria, the Golgi functions and the endoplasmatic reticulum, the nuclear membrane, etc.

Are you a victim of free radical attack?

Do you bruise easily?

Capillary fragility is the result of free radical damage upon the capillaries. Fragile capillaries are prone to leak blood with the slightest bump. You may not even remember how you obtained many bruises because the bump seemed insignificant at the time.

Do you have a lot of wrinkles?

Wrinkles are the result of the breakdown of collagen tissues in the skin. UV radiation causes free radical formation at the skin and rapid depletion of antioxidant supplies at these areas as well.

Do you have heart disease?

Oxidation of Low Density Lipoproteins (LDL) (the "bad" cholesterol) creates free radicals and a chain reaction of events resulting in plaque buildup and clogged arteries.

Do you have arthritis?

The pain and swelling of arthritis is also caused by free radicals which in tissues generate more free radicals and the release of harmful inflammatory prostaglandins.

Do you have cancer?

There are probably over 100 different types of cancer and probably hundreds of ways which free radicals can cause damage associated with cancer. Here are just a few examples.

Carcinogens and many other things such as radiation (including sunlight) form free radicals in the body and can activate oncogenes which cause cancer.

Free radicals can also damage sensors on cell membranes that regulate cell growth and proliferation. If sensors are damaged, unregulated growth can occur. Unregulated growth and cancer go hand in hand.

Free radicals can damage the genetic material (DNA in the nucleus) causing mutation of the cell.

Free radicals can also damage components of the immune system such as white blood cells or enzymes

15

which would otherwise recognize and destroy mutated cells before they multiply and become cancerous.

Do you have cataracts?

The sensitive protein tissues in the eye are highly susceptible to free radical damage if there are inadequate antioxidants to stop the damage. Excess sunlight is a risk factor for cataracts. Free radicals created by sunlight and other factors can also damage the retina, causing retinopathy, or the macular nerve, causing macular degeneration.

Do you have allergies or asthma?

Epidemiological studies show associations among oxidant exposure, respiratory infections, and asthma in children of smokers. Symptoms of ongoing asthma in adults appear to be increased by exposure to environmental oxidants and decreased by antioxidant supplementation. There is evidence that oxidants produced in the body by overactive inflammatory cells contribute to ongoing asthma and allergic hypersensitivities. (Hatch)

Are you aging "prematurely"?

Cellular damage by oxygen radicals is believed to be directly involved in aging, causing the pathological changes associated with aging. The higher the level of free radicals we have in our cells, the faster we age. (Packer)

As we age, we become more susceptible to "age-related diseases" such as diabetes, arthritis, vascular diseases, including coronary artery disease, and hypertension. Interestingly enough, we know now that with antioxidants, these, are all, to some extent, preventable!

Pathological Aspects of Oxidants

Oxygen activation is essential for aerobic life and is involved in numerous vital processes. Keeping these activating reactions under control through detoxification reactions and protective systems is of great importance. A lack of protective or repair capacity results in cell and tissue damage.

Free Radicals Impair Our Immune System

The integrity of the membrane determines its ability to function properly. For example, the phagocyte can only move actively toward an invading bacterium when its cell membrane is intact. Other dependent functions are communication between the cells in tissues and also recognition and identification processes. Our immune system is greatly affected as it is the responsibility of white blood cells to seek out and destroy invaders. If they cannot be identified as harmful, they will not be destroyed and instead will multiply and cause problems.

Some cells, such as a heart muscle cell or a liver cell, may become irreversibly damaged when exposed to oxidative stress. After the membrane structure is disrupted, the cell is no longer able to accomplish its functions. If the damaged cells are not removed by phagocytes, the result may even be malignant transformation of the cell.

The damage produced varies depending on the site of radical attack. Free radicals damage membranes (creating capillary fragility, and associated with cardiovascular disease), damage to ocular lens proteins (creating cataracts), and breakdown of elastin and collagen (associated with aging and wrinkles), and cancer.

With regard to inflammatory, immunoreactive damage, radicals are produced by activated white blood cells (phagocytes). In the case of chronic tissue inflammation, oxygen turnover is increased a hundredfold and tissues are flooded with free radicals.

Free Radicals Destroy Proteins/ DNA

In addition to damaging membranes, protein destruction may also occur which can lead to specific diseases depending on the type of protein. When proteins are affected, metabolic disorders develop, whereas DNA lesions are associated with an increased rate of metagenesis and carcinogenesis. Thus, a broad spectrum of injuries may occur in tissues as a result of enhanced radical formation.

Direct radical attack to the DNA results in an increase in **cancer incidence.** There is sufficient evidence for a relation between free radicals and cancer at least from invitro experiments, animal studies and epidemiologic trials. Cancer is most certainly a "free-radical associated disease."

Free Radicals and Heart Disease

Free radical attack is also directed against plasma lipoproteins and thus plays a role in the development of atherosclerosis. The atherogenic low density lipoprotein (LDL) is a form of cholesterol that has been damaged by oxygen radical attack and thus can no longer be recognized by LDL receptors. It is considered a foreign substance and is attacked by phagocytes. Foam cells are the first sign of an atherosclerotic lesion, representing macrophages which have incorporated oxidized LDL and, through migration into the vessel wall and production of growth factors, produce an early lesion that develops to an atherosclerotic plaque.

INVOLVEMENT OF FREE RADICALS IN HEART DISEASE

| LDL oxidation *

| Macrophages - Uptake by scavenger receptors

| Foam cell formation *

| Fatty streak formation *

| Plaque buildup

| Coronary artery disease

▼ Acute heart failure

Death

Free radical reaction and lipid peroxidation

Free Radicals and Arthritis

The cause and progression of the degenerative processes within joint cavities as in arthritis and osteoarthritis, etc., is due, at least in part, to the destructive activity of oxygen radicals. (Elstner, 1990). Studies (invivo) show that the breakdown of hyaluronic acid by oxygen radicals (OH-) appears to play a role in the loss of function of synovial fluid (joint lubricant). (Peroxinorm) Without this protective fluid to cushion the joints, pain, inflammation and scar tissue develop.

To make things worse, more free radicals are produced by activated phagocytes due to the inflammation. Oxygen turnover is increased in these situations and tissues are literally flooded with free radicals, creating an endless destructive cycle. Therefore, the term "degenerative" is commonly associated with these conditions as the situation progressively worsens.

Free Radicals and Neurological Damage

Nerve tissue is especially susceptible to radical attack because of its high phospholipid content. Additionally, because of the high energy turnover in the brain (cerebrum) and, the extensive oxygen supply required, this tissue is also particularly susceptible to damage. Higher energy requires higher levels of antioxidants to balance the higher level of oxidants produced.

A number of disease conditions are associated with low levels of antioxidants which creates an increased risk for degenerative nerve conditions. A very important group of diseases with increasing significance due to the increasing number of "seniors" in our population are the neurodegenerative disorders, which may be classed under the term "senile dementia." Examples of this include Parkinson's and Alzheimer's diseases.

Oxygen may be activated in the presence of specific heavy metals. Certain transition metals are greatly concentrated in some regions of the brain, and that is why damage to these regions develops so quickly.

Free Radicals and Sugar

High blood sugar levels cause protein damage as the nonenzymatic joining of sugar to protein forms destructive oxygen radicals. The process of forming sugar-damaged proteins is called **glycation**, which can be compared to the browning reaction of sliced apples.

Blood sugar (glucose) and some other sugars react spontaneously with collagen, a major protein found in skin, blood vessels and connective tissue, and other proteins to form cross-linked sugar-damaged proteins. These are called advanced glycosylation end products (AGEs). When these are formed, additional free radicals are released as well. (Tritschler)

The formation rate of AGEs (and free radicals) increases as the blood sugar level increases and the length of time the level is raised increases.

Blood Sugar, Aging and Disease

The spontaneous reaction of sugar with tissue proteins such as collagen and myelin is responsible for accelerated tissue aging in diabetics, is believed responsible for kidney damage, and is also involved in the atherosclerosis process, both common complications of diabetes. Dr. Anthony Cerami observed that glycation reactions also play a role in the normal aging of tissue. This observation led to his glycation hypothesis of aging. Recent studies show that diabetics as well as aging animals do indeed have increased concentrations of AGEs in their collagen.

As we age, our average blood sugar level tends to rise. This is because our tissues become less sensitive to the actions of insulin (insulin resistance) as we get older.

The roles of oxygen and sugar-damaged protein definitely explain much of the secondary aging effects and some of the primary aging process. Maintaining even and optimal blood sugar levels throughout life should protect our tissues from "aging."

Antioxidants and Antiglycation

Both free radical reduction and glycation reduction reduce the incidence of the aging diseases, including heart disease, arthritis and cancer. They are complimentary approaches that enhance each other's benefits. The protection against free-radical damage is more efficient with both approaches than through the actions of either alone.

Some cellular damage caused by radicals can be repaired by enzymes. We actually produce some enzymes in the body for the sole purpose of repairing damage to cells caused by radicals and by high levels of blood sugar. However, adequate levels of antioxidants are needed to protect these enzymes from free radical damage as well.

Cellular Protection Systems

Our cells do not lack protection against free radicals. Protection and repair systems are available which, within their capacity limits, allow oxygen activation to occur with no resulting damage. Among these protection systems are enzymes like superoxide dismutase (SOD), catalase, peroxidases or glutathione peroxidase. In addition, in plants as well as in animals, there are metabolites such as ascorbic acid (Vitamin C), α-tocopherol (Vitamin E), sulphur-containing amino acids like cysteine and glutathione, and various carotenoids, odiphenoles and sugars which act as radical scavengers.

The goal is to obtain a balance between oxidants and antioxidants in the body. If you have more oxidants than you do antioxidants, the result is damage to the cells, tissues, etc. On the other hand, if the level of antioxidants in the body is higher than the level of free radicals, the excess antioxidants may actually create free radicals.

In Search of
The Perfect Antioxidant

Supplemental antioxidants are useful to keep free radicals in check and to maintain good health. Although there is no one, single, perfect antioxidant, α–lipoic acid is a candidate which approaches that ideal. The antioxidant nutrients are partners working together. Vitamins C, E and A are essential vitamins as well as antioxidants. However, they all work better when α–lipoic acid is available in levels where it can be used as an antioxidant, not merely tied up as a coenzyme.

Dr. Lester Packer, Professor at the University of California, Berkeley, Department of Molecular and Cell Biology, is among the world's leading antioxidant researchers, and is perhaps the foremost researcher on α–Lipoic Acid. He has described an ideal antioxidant as one that has the following biochemical properties:

1) quenches a variety of oxidative species

2) is easily absorbed and is readily bioavailable

3) exists in a variety of locations: tissues, cells, extracellular fluid, intracellular fluid, various membranes, etc.

4) interacts with other antioxidants

5) chelates free metal ions

6) has positive effects on gene expression

α–Lipoic Acid and DHLA (the reduced form of α–Lipoic Acid) do all of the above very well.

23

α–Lipoic Acid: The Ideal Antioxidant

α–Lipoic Acid is the ideal antioxidant because it is both water and fat soluble, works inside and outside of cells, participates in redox cycling by breaking down to Dihydrolipoic Acid (DHLA) which recharges other important antioxidants and quenches several free radicals and reactive oxygen species. Together the team is effective against almost all species of radicals.

α–Lipoic Acid terminates the hydroxyl and hypochlorous free radicals. Its reduced form, DHLA, terminates hydroxyl and hypochlorous free radicals and, in addition, terminates superoxide free radicals and peroxyl free radicals. α–Lipoic Acid also quenches the reactive oxygen species singlet oxygen and possibly hydrogen peroxide in some domains but not in others.

α–Lipoic Acid can partially replace some of the dietary need for Vitamins C and E. In 1959, Drs. Rosenberg and Culik showed that α–Lipoic Acid prevented scurvy in Vitamin C-deficient animals, and that it prevented symptoms of Vitamin E deficiency in laboratory animals fed a Vitamin E-deficient diet. They even predicted that α–Lipoic Acid might act as an antioxidant for Vitamins C and E.

What Makes α-Lipoic Acid Special?

1. The structure of α–Lipoic Acid is very small, which allows it to slip through cell membranes providing antioxidant protection on both the inside and outside of cells. Most antioxidants like Vitamins C and E are too large to pass through the cell membrane and thus offer only protection on the outside of the cell.

2. α–Lipoic Acid possesses antioxidant properties in its original form **and also** in its reduced form, DHLA. α–Lipoic Acid is readily converted to DHLA after being

24

Name	Terminated by α–Lipoic Acid	Terminated by Dihydrolipoic Acid
Superoxide (O2)	No	?
Hydroxy radical (HO)	Yes	Yes
Peroxyl radical (ROO)	Possibly	Possibly
Hypochlorous radical (HOCL)	Yes	Yes
Singlet oxygen	Yes	Yes
Hydrogen peroxide (H2O2)	No	No
Heavy Metals (FE, Cu, Cd, Pb, HG)	Chelated*	Chelated*

Chelation refers to the ability to "chelate" or grab hold of metallic substances that might otherwise cause toxicity.

ingested as a supplement.

Most antioxidant substances can act as antioxidants only in their reduced forms. After they have donated an electron, they are then "used up" unless they are regenerated by another antioxidant (like α–Lipoic Acid).

3. In its oxidized form, surface atoms at the end of the molecule form a ring structure known as the dithiole ring. (A disulfide molecule located in this ring allows α–Lipoic Acid to act as an enzyme catalyst.) When this ring is broken, either through oxidation or through enzymes, the result is dihydrolipoic Acid (DHLA) which is an even more potent antioxidant than α–Lipoic Acid.

4. α–Lipoic Acid has functions in the body besides its antioxidant activities. α–Lipoic Acid is first a coenzyme in the metabolic process and is necessary for the conversion of glucose to energy (ATP). Small amounts of Lipoic Acid are bound chemically at the active sites of enzymes. Second, when higher levels are achieved in the body through supplementation, it acts as a potent antioxidant.

25

α-Lipoic Acid Recycles

When an antioxidant such as Vitamin E donates an electron to a radical, the Vitamin E is oxidized and the radical is reduced. If the Vitamin E does not receive another electron from another molecule, it is used up. If the Vitamin E is reduced, it recycles back to its original form.

Lipoic Acid has a very low redox potential. This means that in its reduced form (DHLA), it very readily donates electrons to either stabilize a radical or recycle an oxidized molecule (like Vitamin E). Thus, α-Lipoic Acid can not only terminate free radicals, but it can also regenerate other antioxidants in the body allowing them to continue to scavenge free radicals.

The body produces enzymes (superoxide dismutase, glutathione peroxidase, and catalase) which protect us from free radical damage. We can also help protect ourselves through ingesting foods containing high amounts of antioxidants or by supplementing nutrients such as ascorbic acid, α-tocopherol or the carotenoids. Other nutrients are also required for the body to either manufacture these substances or to utilize them. These include zinc, copper, manganese in the case of superoxide dismutase, or selenium and cysteine in the case of glutathione peroxidase.

Significance of Glutathione

Glutathione (from the amino acid glutamic acid) plays an important role in cell detoxification, DNA and protein synthesis, transport processes and in the removal of oxidants.

Glutathione peroxidase not only eliminates hydrogen peroxide but it also repairs damage which has already occurred. Following the oxidation of fatty acids to hydroperoxides, glutathione peroxidase prevents this activity from continuing any further. It is a true repair enzyme for membrane lesions. Ascorbic acid, α–tocopherol, and the carotenoids can reduce free radicals directly by sacrificing an electron.

Glutathione synthesis in the body is dependent upon the intracellular availability of the essential amino acid cysteine. Lester Packer has reported that administration of α–Lipoic Acid is beneficial in several oxidative stress situations probably because of an increase in cellular glutathione content. (Packer and Busse) Just recently, however, German researchers demonstrated that this is due to an enhanced cysteine supply following administration of DHLA. (Kis)

♦ Glutathione in both its oxidized and reduced form functions very similarly to the manner in which Lipoic Acid/DHLA functions.

♦ Glutamic acid passes the blood brain barrier and is considered "brain fuel." It is necessary for a healthy brain and a healthy attitude, too!

♦ Glutamic acid gives rise to GABA (a calming agent in the brain) and possibly to neurotransmitters.

♦ Glutamic acid is a component of folic acid.

♦ Glutamic acid and also cysteine are necessary for glucose regulation.

♦ Glutamic acid and cysteine protect against the effects of alcohol and smoking. Glutamic acid can also decrease cravings for alcohol and sometimes, sugar.

♦ Cysteine is necessary for production of glutathione in the body.

♦ Cysteine removes heavy metal deposits.

♦ Cysteine production in the body is inhibited by chronic illness.

27

Low levels of glutathione and cysteine associated with health problems

Reduced levels of glutathione (as well as a number of other antioxidants) are seen among individuals with many health problems. These include:

Diabetes	Cardiovascular Disease
HIV	Chronic Fatigue
Asthma	Osteoporosis
Allergies	Kidney Disease
Arthritis	Lupus
Alcoholism	*(also, chronic crankiness!)*

α-Lipoic Acid Increases Glutathione Levels

As part of its regeneration of its partner antioxidant, α–Lipoic Acid also increases cellular glutathione content. Glutathione is a major antioxidant within cells and glutathione peroxidase is the major repair enzyme.

Glutathione and α-Lipoic Acid Regenerate E

In a low density lipoprotein (LDL) which consists of about 1,300 molecules, there are about 7.5 moles of antioxidants (mostly α-tocopherol) per LDL molecule, depending on one's diet and other factors.

Membranes possess many double bonds, and radical chain reactions may easily be initiated under the influence of oxygen, leading to an oxidation process that sweeps across the membrane.

To stop the chain reaction, some kinds of "radical extinguishers" are incorporated in the membrane:

28

for instance, Vitamin E. The radical chain reaction ends at the place on the membrane where a Vitamin E molecule is situated.

When Vitamin E is oxidized, its protective activity is lost. Regeneration of the E molecule can occur through glutathione peroxidase and ascorbic acid, but as they do so, they too are oxidized and used up.

Obviously, increasing the amount of Vitamin E would protect us against damage. If α–Lipoic Acid, glutathione and Vitamin C are present, they have a synergistic effect to protect against the loss of Vitamin E. This means that it takes longer for the free radicals to damage the molecule.

α-Lipoic Acid/DHLA Work with C and E

The direct free radical scavenging effect of DHLA is not the only mode of its antioxidant action. DHLA can also synergistically enhance antioxidant protective activity of membranes by recycling tocopherol radicals and working synergistically with Vitamin C. (Bast and Haenen; Scholich)

DHLA can bolster the antioxidant systems by interacting with other redox couples (Packer, 1989; Kagan, Maguire) and LDL. (Kagan, Freisleben, Kagan, Serbinova)

Dr. Packer reports that the research he has done leaves little doubt about the antioxidant effectiveness of DHLA which can directly scavenge peroxyl and superoxide radicals and/or enhance other water- or lipid-soluble antioxidants (ascorbate, Vitamin E) by regenerating them via the reduction of their radicals.

The Lipoic Acid/DHLA redox couple has been found to exert a synergistic action in the antioxidant recycling mechanisms of natural membranes and LDL in vitro and in protecting against oxidative injury.

29

EXPOSURE TO AN OXIDANT ⟶	LOSS OF E
If no protection is added:	**100%**
If dihydrolipoate is added:	90%
If ascorbate (vitamin C) is added:	60%
If both C and dihydrolipoate are added:	**30%**

(Packer, *The Vitamin E, Ascorbate and α–lipoate Antioxidant Defense System...*)

When antioxidants have a high affinity for certain free radicals they are recognized as part of the **thiol antioxidant system**. Glutathione is also part of this system as dihydrolipoate has a similar recycling effect on glutathione. Lipoic Acid is also known as **Thiotic Acid.**

One can predict that protection should be increased by bolstering antioxidant defenses. Researchers have tested this hypothesis and demonstrated that Lipoic Acid supplementation protects tissues in organs such as the liver, heart, brain, and skin against lipid peroxidation induced by peroxyl radicals.

Because of the association of disease with the significant damage to membrane phospholipids from free radical peroxidation, researchers are feverishly examining the antioxidant effects of Lipoic Acid and DHLA. (Bast, Scholich, Muller, Bonomi, DeMascio)

However, the results of these experiments are controversial. Some researchers have reported that neither DHLA nor Lipoic Acid themselves protect against microsomal lipid peroxidation induced by iron + ascorbate. There also is concern that DHLA may create free radicals as a pro-oxidant (probably due to the reduction of iron). The protective antioxidant effect was detected only when the combination of DHLA and oxidized glutathione was present. (Bast, Prujin)

What does this mean? It means we don't have all the answers, but it also may be an indication that too much of a good thing, may no longer be beneficial and may actually be detrimental.

α-Lipoic Acid Prevents Glycation

Lipoic Acid effectively reduces the protein damage that high blood sugar levels cause. With α–Lipoic Acid's antiglycation action to prevent the damage from blood sugar, and its antioxidant action to protect against free radicals, the minor damage that does occur can be repaired by the still-functioning enzymes. The result is that the cell is protected and the body does not become damaged and thereby one cell older.

DHLA: Both Fat and Water Soluble

Lipoic Acid alone is not effective in scavenging all types of free radicals. For example, α–Lipoic Acid is not effective against peroxyl radicals. However, it readily converts to DHLA in the body which can usually effectively ward off damage from these radicals as it can function as a radical scavenger against both water-soluble and lipid-soluble radicals. This is the only known antioxidant which has this special property of acting in both water and fat soluble mediums.

Since transition metals were not used for peroxyl radical generation, these effects cannot be caused by chelation of transition metals. There is no requirement for either Vitamin E or glutathione to display this direct anti radical activity of DHLA. Thus, in contrast to many other antioxidants, DHLA may function as a universal free radical quencher which can scavenge radicals in areas where other antioxidants cannot.

31

α-Lipoic Acid: Therapeutic Uses

Lipoic Acid is currently used as a therapeutic agent in a variety of diseases, including liver and neurological disorders. Patients diagnosed with liver cirrhosis, diabetes, atherosclerosis and polyneuritis have been found to contain a reduced level of α–Lipoic Acid in the body. (Altenkirch, Piering)

Inside the cell, DHLA, is even more potent than α–Lipoic Acid in performing antioxidant functions. DHLA directly destroys damaging superoxide radicals, hydroperoxy radicals and hydroxyl radicals.

In order to perform this antioxidant function in the body, α-Lipoic Acid must be present in amounts significantly higher than normal. Therefore, supplementation is required for this great benefit to be obtained. 100 to 200 mg. daily is sufficient to obtain antioxidant benefits. Therapeutic doses may be higher. Some studies use daily dosages as high as 600 and 800 mg. Side effects even at this dosage are practically non-existent. No toxic effects have been reported with the exception of some concern of its action as a pro-oxidant under certain circumstances.

Cancer and α-Lipoic Acid

Cancer is the result of external factors combined with a genetic disposition for cancer, usually localized. Research data indicate that free radicals are involved in the process of cancer initiation and promotion.

As mentioned earlier, there are probably over 100 different ways in which free radicals can cause damage associated with cancer. Carcinogens and many other things such as radiation (including sunlight) which form free radicals in the body can activate oncogenes which cause cancer.

Free radicals can also damage sensors on cell membranes that regulate cell growth and proliferation. If sensors are damaged, unregulated growth can occur. Unregulated growth and cancer go hand in hand.

Free radicals can damage the genetic material (DNA in the nucleus), causing mutation of the cell.

Free radicals can also damage the immune system which would otherwise recognize and destroy mutated cells before they multiply and become cancerous.

Protection of Genetic Material

Lipoic Acid plays a major role in protecting the genes that determine our health. We know that our family history (our genetics) can increase our susceptibility to certain diseases such as breast cancer, colon cancer, melanoma, etc. As long as we can prevent this gene from activation, it won't cause any problem. We can do this if certain antioxidants prevent free radicals from reaching the gene.

A gene is a segment of DNA that operates as a unit within a chromosome to control a specific cell function. There are about 100,000 genes in each of the 46 chromosomes in the nucleus of cells. Genes can reproduce themselves at each cell division, and manage the formation of body proteins through processes called gene expression and regulation. Free radicals and other reactive oxygen species which interfere with normal gene regulation can profoundly influence health and life span.

Genes can be activated by a protein complex within the cell called Nuclear Factor kappa–B (NF-kappa–B). Oxidation can activate NF-kappa–B causing it bind to DNA in genes and initiate reproduction. As we grow older, we have higher amounts of activated NF-kappa–B bound to our genes than we did when we were younger.

NF-kappa–B has a negative effect on the immune system, and can also cause defective skin cells and aged skin, defective cells in all organs impairing function of all body systems.

Free radicals, peroxides, and ultraviolet energy can induce the inactive complex to dissociate and allow the NF-kappa–B to penetrate into the nucleus and damage DNA.

Antioxidants Keep NF-kappa–B in Check

The action of NF-kappa–B is controlled by protein sub-units called I-kappa–B proteins. When an I-kappa–B protein binds to NF-kappa–B, the complex cannot pass from the cell cytoplasm through the porous two-layered membrane of the nuclear envelope into the nucleus where the genes are located. The goal for health is to prevent the release of excess NF-kappa–B from the complex, and to permit the body to control its release by normal processes.

Antioxidants inhibit free radicals and other reactive oxygen species and are therefore able to inhibit this activation. Lipoic Acid is of particular interest because of its ability to work inside the cell. As a relatively very small molecule, it is readily transported through cellular membranes, including the nuclear membrane. It can therefore not only terminate free radicals in the bloodstream and on the cellular membrane, but it can also protect NF kappa–B inside the cell from activation and protect the DNA and genes from damage from certain nuclear factors.

α-Lipoic Acid Protects Skin from Cancer and Aging

Skin, as the outermost barrier of the body, is constantly exposed to a variety of oxidative stresses and injury. Topical application of antioxidants is one way to diminish oxidative injury. Lipoic Acid, as a potent antioxidant with both fat- and water-soluble properties, makes it an excellent candidate for antioxidant protection for the skin.

Skin cells will convert and release about 25% of the α–Lipoic Acid to DHLA. UV radiation is known to deplete the lipophilic antioxidants tocopherol and ubiquinol in skin. α–Lipoic Acid was found to significantly protect UV-light induced depletion of ubiquinol by 40% if topically applied 2 hours prior to irradiation. (Podda)

α–Lipoic Acid and DHLA protect against induced lipid peroxidation and appear to protect special fat-soluble antioxidants in the body which protect our skin. After administration of Lipoic Acid to female hairless mice for seven weeks, it was observed that

35

the major antioxidant levels in the skin increased.

UV radiation (both A and B gamma rays) is known to cause drastic depletion of these fat-soluble antioxidants. In the Lipoic Acid-fed animals, some sparing against the loss of these antioxidants occurred. At the end of the irradiation period in the Lipoic Acid-administered animals, the levels of antioxidants, such as α–tocopherol, ubiquinols and ubiquinones (i.e., Co-Q10), were higher than in the skin of controls.

Collagen damage due to oxidative damage in the skin increases between 30 to 40% after exposure to UVAB radiation. The degree of damage was lower in the skin of the Lipoic Acid-fed animals both before and after UV radiation. These findings have important implications for skin cancer and skin diseases since depletion of the antioxidant defense mechanism in the skin leads to molecular damage. (Reznick, Witt, and Packer)

- - - - = denotes baseline	Exposure to UV Radiation W/O α–Lipoic Acid supplementation	Exposure to UV Radiation WITH α–Lipoic Acid supplementation
Free radicals	↗	↗
α-Lipoic Acid	↘	↗
Vitamin E	↘	→
Other antioxidants	↘	→
Collagen Damage	↗	→

α-Lipoic Acid Prevents Radiation Damage

Irradiation is known to produce a cascade of free radicals, and antioxidant compounds have long been used to treat irradiation injury. Lipoic Acid, but not DHLA, has demonstrated protective effects against radiation injury to sensitive tissues in the body such as the liver where cells are slow to replace themselves. (Ramakrishnan, Kropachova)

The potential benefit of this effect is not only for individuals undergoing irradiation treatment for cancer, but for all of us who are exposed to radiation from the sun. We know that radiation hastens aging of the skin and increases our risk for cataracts, but it is likely to also cause damage in other areas of the body. It would be almost impossible to do studies for every potential protective benefit of α–Lipoic Acid on every area of the body.

α-Lipoic Acid Increases Glutathione

In vitro studies demonstrated a dose-dependent increase of 30 to 70% of the glutathione content following Lipoic Acid administration.

Normal lung tissue of mice also revealed about 50% increase in glutathione upon treatment with α–Lipoic Acid. This corresponds with protection from irradiation damage in these in vitro studies. (Busse)

Human Studies Confirm Protective Effects of α-Lipoic Acid

A recent study examined the effects of 28 days of antioxidant treatment on a variety of blood and urinary parameters in children living in areas affected by the Chernobyl nuclear accident who are continuously exposed to low-level radiation.

37

♦ Treatment with α–Lipoic Acid alone lowered blood peroxidation values to the same level seen in non-radiation-exposed children.

♦ Treatment with α–Lipoic Acid with Vitamin E further lowered blood peroxidation to below-normal values. Vitamin E alone was without effect.

♦ Urinary excretion of radioactive metabolites was also lowered by α–Lipoic Acid but not by Vitamin E, presumably due to chelation by α–Lipoic Acid.

♦ Liver and kidney functions were also normalized by α–Lipoic Acid treatment. (Korina)

α-Lipoic Acid and Inflammatory Conditions

Oxidants produced in the body by overactive inflammatory cells, phagocytes, macrophages and other white blood cells can increase free radicals by a hundredfold and flood tissue, causing localized damage.

Allergies and Antioxidants

Individuals with hypersensitivities are highly susceptible to overactive inflammatory cell activity. The T-suppressor cell is the most sensitive cell of the immune system and the first to be affected by exposure to chemical free radical pollutants. (Most people don't realize that many substances which irritate allergies (cigarette smoke, smog, pesticides, etc.) are free radicals.) Diminishment of the T-suppressor activity, in turn, increases T-helper cell activity which leads to increased immunoglobulin production and the manifestation of allergy symptoms.

Allergies are difficult to treat because each exposure to the offending substances further weakens the system, with the creation of even more free radicals. Removal of these chemical pollutants from the body as quickly as possible is essential for effective treatment of this problem. Dietary antioxidants help reduce the oxidizing effect of the pollutants and act as conjugators to remove the pollutants from the body. (Trevino)

Asthma and Antioxidants

In the last decade we have seen numerous reports of the increased number of asthmatics and asthmatic children. There also has been an increase in the number of asthma-related deaths, in spite of medical advances. Higher levels of free radicals due to our industrialized world may be directly correlated.

Asthmatics have a higher level of free radical production which is generated by decreased circulating platelets (red blood cells) and higher levels of white blood cells (neutrophils and macrophages) compared to non-asthmatics. Platelets are natural inhibitors of the free-radical processes in non-asthmatic individuals. In asthmatic patients the free-radical-inhibitory function of platelets decreases.

Antioxidants help normalize platelets in asthmatics by decreasing the presence of white blood cells (neutrophils and macrophages) which are sent in by the body's defense system to combat the "invader" cat dander, pollen, mold, etc.

Asthma attacks spur free radical production

Oxygen-derived radicals play key roles in allergic inflammatory responses in asthma. These radicals produce many of the pathophysiologic changes associated with asthma and may contribute to its pathogenesis.

Researchers showed that following a severe asthma attack the number of white blood cells in lung fluid was increased 3.5 fold compared with nonsensitized but challenged control animals. They also found that the presence of lipid peroxidation products was 2.4 times higher compared to the controls.

Antioxidant levels were far **lower** in the lung fluid of the sensitized, challenged animals. The concentration of Vitamin E, the major lipid-soluble antioxidant, was 8.7 times lower than that in nonsensitized controls and the reserve of water-soluble antioxidants (thiols and ascorbic acid) was 4 times lower than controls. This indicates an antioxidant/pro-oxidant imbalance associated with an asthmatic episode. (Shvedoda)

Free radicals cause bronchoconstriction, increase mucus and swelling

Researchers in The Netherlands showed how pulmonary tissue can be damaged in different ways by free radicals formed during inflammation, ischemia reperfusion, or exposure to irritants.

The reactive oxygen species induce bronchoconstriction, elevate mucus secretion, and cause microvascular leakage, which leads to edema. Reactive oxygen species even induce an autonomic imbalance between muscarinic receptor mediated contraction and the beta–adrenergic-mediated relaxation of the pulmonary smooth muscle.

Vitamin E and selenium have a regulatory role in this balance between these two receptor responses. The autonomic imbalance might be involved in the development of bronchial hyper-responsiveness, occurring in lung inflammation. (Doelman)

Glutathione levels reduced in asthmatics

Reduced levels of glutathione peroxidase have been observed in adults and children with asthma in several studies. (Powell, Novak)

The Novak antioxidant study revealed the impact of asthma on glutathione and the proportion of hemoglobin oxidation products in children. A decreased catalase enzyme activity and a significantly reduced glutathione instability were demonstrated as compared to the controls. The results indicate that antioxidant protection of hemoglobin in asthmatic children is considerably decreased. Hemoglobin is a

41

protein-iron compound in the blood which carries oxygen to the tissues. (Novak)

Antioxidants Lessen Damage Caused by Free Radicals

Antioxidants can inhibit the damage caused by these free radicals. (Smith)

Vitamin C intake in the general population appears to correlate with incidence for asthma, suggesting that a diet low in Vitamin C is a risk factor for asthma. Studies also show the harmful effects of free radical exposure in children of smokers, resulting in respiratory infections and asthma. Symptoms of ongoing asthma in adults appear to be increased by exposure to environmental oxidants and decreased by Vitamin C supplementation. There is evidence that oxidants produced in the body by overactive inflammatory cells contribute to ongoing asthma.

Vitamin C is the major antioxidant substance present in the airway surface liquid of the lung, where it can protect against oxidants produced within the body as well as environmental oxidants. Nitrogen oxides are oxidants that could arise from both endogenous and environmental sources, which are protected against by Vitamin C, and may be important in the causation and propagation of asthma. (Hatch)

Platelet Abnormalities Reduced

Thirty healthy controls and 37 asthmatic patients were observed to determine the effects of platelets on the free radical generation by neutrophils and macrophages and on lipid peroxidation. In healthy individuals, blood plasma poor in platelets

(PPP) induced a higher production of free radicals compared to plasma rich in platelets (PRP).

The results obtained in healthy donors demonstrated the inhibitory effect of platelets on free radical generation in asthmatic patients, as compared to healthy donors where the inhibitory effect of platelets on free radical generation decreases 1.3 - 1.2 times.

Antioxidant supplementation inhibited platelets both on free radical (1.4 times) and on lipid peroxidation (1.3 times) and a more marked decrease of neutrophils (1.4 times) compared to patients who did not receive supplementation. The antioxidant preparation potentiates platelet function and accordingly decreases the level of free radicals in blood which prevents inflammation and bronchoconstriction. (Boljevic)

Number of Free Radicals Reduced

A study was made of the generation of active forms of oxygen by leukocytes and of the free radical lipid peroxidation and antiperoxide activity in 52 bronchial asthma patients in relation to supplementation with antioxidants. In bronchial asthma exacerbation, free radical production increases compared to the control.

During remission, free radical production decreases but does not reach normal. Bronchial asthma patients receiving antioxidants in addition to the conventional therapy demonstrated a more pronounced lowering of free radical production than those given the conventional therapy alone, providing evidence in favor of including antioxidants in combined therapy of bronchial asthma. (Daniliak)

Other studies have also demonstrated this beneficial effect of antioxidants. Boljevic found that in patients with steroid-dependent bronchial asthma, the free radical process is more intensive. Regarding the free radical process the most responsive to antioxidant supplementation was aspirin asthma, the mildest exercise-induced asthma. In patients with steroid-non-dependent bronchial asthma and in patients with steroid-dependent bronchial asthma receiving traditional therapy and antioxidants (Vitamins E and A and glutamic acid), the decreased free radical generation and decreased effects were greater than in patients not taking antioxidants. (Boljevic)

α-Lipoic Acid and Asthma

Because of what we have already seen α–Lipoic Acid is capable of, these studies demonstrate the need for α–Lipoic Acid supplementation which not only regenerates Vitamins E and C, but also increases glutathione levels.

Antioxidants decrease inflammation

A study to compare the effects of several different antioxidants, including a thiol group, on individuals with bronchial asthma was conducted. They examined respiratory function, hydroperoxides, total and non-protein thiol groups, and inflammatory and anti-inflammatory prostaglandins. All antioxidants were found to lower hydroperoxides (free radicals) and increase the content of thiol groups (group of antioxidants which includes glutathione and α–Lipoic Acid). The researchers noted a rise in the level of anti-inflammatory prostaglandins and a considerable reduction of inflammatory prostaglandins after antioxidant administration. (Amatuni) Increased thiol antioxidants were found to decrease free radicals and reduce inflammatory prostaglandins.

44

Arthritis

Oxygen free radicals cause tissue degeneration in joint cavities (arthritis, osteoarthritis). The decomposition of hyaluronic acid by free radicals appears to play a role in vivo in the oxidative loss of function of synovial fluid (joint lubricant).

Researchers are now investigating the potential benefit of antioxidant substances for oxygen radicals with inflammatory associated processes of rheumatic joint disease. For example, several studies have demonstrated antioxidants (1,200 mg. α–tocopherol) to be safe and effective against arthritis to help improve mobility, reduce pain and reduce need for additional analgesic medication. (Packer)

The fact that OH- radicals can be generated via intermediate formation of superoxide may explain the improvement observed after intra-articular administration of superoxide dismutase. (Peroxinorm)

Low Antioxidant Levels are a Risk Factor for Arthritis

Several micronutrients acting as antioxidants and free radical scavengers have demonstrated protective effects against rheumatoid arthritis.

A case control 20 year study was nested within a Finnish group of 1,419 adult men and women. Fourteen of the individuals who were initially free of arthritis developed rheumatoid arthritis. Serum α–tocopherol, β-carotene and selenium concentrations were compared.

Elevated risks of rheumatoid arthritis were observed at low levels of α–tocopherol, β–carotene and selenium demonstrating that a low antioxidant level is a risk factor for rheumatoid arthritis. (Heliovaara)

45

Significance of Glutathione

The reactive oxygen radicals are trapped by antioxidants such as selenium containing glutathione peroxidase, which also can inhibit the oxygenation of arachidonic acid to inflammatory prostaglandins and leukotrienes. (Honkanen)

Iron Oxidation Aggravates Inflammatory Problems

Researchers in London point out the need for adequate antioxidant levels to protect us from the potential harmful effects of iron oxidation. Iron is an essential mineral involved in the transport of oxygen, in electron transfer, in the synthesis of DNA, in oxidations by oxygen (O_2) and hydrogen peroxide (H_2O_2), and in many other processes necessary to maintain normal structure and function of virtually all mammalian cells.

However, without adequate antioxidants to keep iron oxidation from causing damage, iron oxidation aggravates inflammation through the generation of reactive oxygen intermediates and also through the developments of additional free radicals, including the reaction of iron with nitric oxide.

Iron oxidation also increases damage associated with hypoxia-reperfusion injury (heart attack and stroke) and diseases of the skin (such as psoriasis abd allergic hives) and joint (such as arthritis and osteoarthritis). (Morris)

Osteoarthritis

Osteoarthritis, like rheumatoid arthritis, is an age-related disease, in which degenerative changes (arthrosis) and superimposed inflammatory reactions (arthritis) lead to progressive destruction of the joints. Cumulative damage to tissues, mediated by reactive oxygen species, has been implicated as a pathway that leads to many of the degenerative changes associated with aging. Appropriate treatment with antioxidants and free radical scavengers is recommended. (Henrotin)

Researchers hypothesized that increased intake of antioxidant micronutrients might be associated with decreased rates of osteoarthritis in the knees. Six hundred forty participants received complete assessments.

A three-fold reduction in risk of osteoarthritis progression was found for both the middle level and highest level of Vitamin C intake. This directly related to a reduced risk of cartilage loss. Those with high Vitamin C intake also had a reduced risk of developing knee pain. A reduction in the risk of osteoarthritis progression was also seen for individuals with an increased β–carotene and Vitamin E intake. (McAlindon)

Psoriasis

Individuals with psoriasis (an inflammatory skin condition) also have lower levels of antioxidants. Chronic inflammation, as we already discussed, greatly stimulates the production of free radicals which can further aggravate almost any health situation.

Red blood cell fatty acid composition and

micronutrient status were investigated in patients with psoriatic arthritis. Red blood cell fatty acid composition, selenium status, red blood cell glutathione-peroxidase activity, plasma levels of copper, zinc, Vitamins A and E, and thiobarbiturate reactive substances where investigated after exposure to an oxidant (H_2O_2). These levels served as an index of susceptibility to lipoperoxidation for 25 patients with psoriatic arthritis and in 25 sex and age matched controls.

Results showed that there was a lower level of the antioxidant selenium in patients with psoriatic arthritis in comparison with controls. Significant direct correlations were observed between red blood cell fatty acids and erythrocyte sedimentation rate, duration of disease and morning stiffness. (Azzini)

This suggests that antioxidant supplementation may benefit individuals with psoriasis.

Sjogren's Disease

Researchers have also determined that patients with Sjogren's Disease may benefit from antioxidant protection from α-Lipoic Acid. Sjogren's Disease is a condition which the eyes, mouth, and vagina become excessively dry. It commonly accompanies auto-immune disorders such as arthritis and Lupus.

Individuals with Sjogren's Disease suffer free radical damage (in the acinar cells basal membranes) due to inadequate antioxidant enzyme systems caused by lipid peroxidation reactions. (Ron)

48

Diabetes and α-Lipoic Acid

Diabetes strikes one of every 20 Americans. Not only is it the third leading cause of death in the U.S., but it also inflicts serious suffering in the form of blindness, nerve damage, heart disease, gangrene, and loss of limbs. In the last 25 years, the incidence of diabetes has increased over 600%, accounting for 300,000 to 350,000 deaths each year during the early 1990s. About half of those with coronary artery disease and three-fourths of those suffering strokes developed their circulatory problems prematurely as a result of diabetes.

Diabetes involves the body's inability to properly metabolize food into energy. The result is a build-up of blood sugar that causes a number of serious problems. With modern-day technology, individuals are able to some degree to self-regulate blood sugar through home glucose tests, medication and insulin. But even so, normal glucose levels for a diabetic (180-250 mg./deciliter) are almost twice the normal range (80-120 mg./deciliter).

The long-term effects of these elevated blood sugar levels result in oxidative damage (glycation) causing diabetic complications such as cataracts, retinopathy, macular degeneration, stiffened arteries and heart tissue via damaged lipoproteins (LDL) and nerve destruction (polyneuropathy). High sugar levels can also result in osmotic changes and reduced blood volume, shock acidosis, coma and death.

49

Insulin-dependent diabetes mellitus (Type I) normally results when the body does not produce enough insulin. This is normally the result of damage to the beta cells of the pancreas. This form of diabetes usually, but not always, begins in childhood; thus it is often referred to as juvenile diabetes.

Non-insulin-dependent diabetes (Type II) accounts for about 85% of diabetes cases and is usually associated with age and/or obesity. It is sometimes called adult-onset diabetes. This form is caused by insulin resistance of cells or the inability of insulin receptors to utilize insulin efficiently. Usually, diet and oral medication can keep blood sugar levels near normal, but insulin is generally of no value. Type II diabetics generally have high levels of insulin in the blood, but it is ineffective because of the insulin resistance of the tissues.

NADH - Antioxidant Levels Lower in Diabetics

NADH (an enzyme involved in the mitrochondrial production of ATP) is the final acceptor of the electrons and thus an appropriate NADH supply is essential for allowing redox reactions to proceed.

In diabetic individuals where huge amounts of NADH are used for the reduction of glucose to sorbitol in non-insulin-dependent tissues, the detoxification processes may be reduced to a clinically significant extent. This is one of the reasons antioxidant levels are so low in diabetics as they are used up rapidly, resulting in extensive free radical damage throughout the body.

α-Lipoic Acid Levels Lower in Diabetics

Patients diagnosed with diabetes and many of the complications associated with diabetes such as polyneuritis and atherosclerosis have been found to have lower levels of endogenous (produced in the body) lipoic acid. (Altnkirch, 1990, Piering, 1990) Because higher levels of free radical damage of membrane phospholipids has been shown to be a characteristic of these conditions, there is a great potential benefit of lipoic acid supplementation.

α-Lipoic Acid Benefits Diabetes I and II

Lipoic Acid has potential beneficial effects for both types of diabetes. Most Type II diabetics are hyperinsulinemic; hence, no insulin therapy is warranted. A number of studies have therefore examined other means of increasing glucose uptake. Agents that enhance glucose uptake by skeletal muscles are potentially useful in the long-term treatment of Type II diabetes. Both human and animal studies show that α–Lipoic Acid enhances glucose utilization. Using the obese Zucker rat as an animal model of insulin resistance in obesity, α–Lipoic Acid treatment increased the uptake of glucose in the absence or presence of insulin in muscles by over 50%. (Henricksen)

Human Studies

In human studies, 1,000 mg. of α–Lipoic Acid administered intravenously to diabetics enhanced insulin-stimulated whole body glucose disposal by about 50%. (Jacob) Supplemental α–Lipoic Acid may bring levels of α–Lipoic Acid in the body, which are known to be low, back to normal. The various beneficial effects of α–Lipoic Acid for diabetics may be due to its reaction with cellular sulfflydryl groups, believed to be involved in the regulation of insulin-stimulated glucose transport. The effect may also be due to the antioxidant function of α–Lipoic Acid. (Packer)

51

α-Lipoic Acid Lowers/Normalizes Blood Sugar Levels

Lipoic Acid not only normalizes blood sugar levels in diabetics; it also protects against the damage responsible for diabetes in the first place. It has been successfully used in Germany for more than 30 years where it has reduced the secondary effects of diabetes, including damage to the retina, cataract formation, nerve and heart damage, as well as increasing energy levels. Lipoic Acid improves nerve blood flow, reduces oxidative stress, and improves distal nerve conduction in diabetic neuropathy.

Lipoic Acid can terminate free radicals and thus reduce the oxidative stress that can damage the pancreas, cause cataracts, nerve damage, retinopathy and other side effects. Lipoic Acid also reduces glycation, which otherwise can damage proteins, especially those of skin and blood vessels. Even more important to diabetics is that α–Lipoic Acid, by virtue of its ability to normalize blood sugar level and the entire glycolysis pathway for conversion of sugar into energy, allows the nerves to recover. Pain is reduced and normal feeling is restored.

Lipoic Acid increases glucose transport by stimulating the glucose transporters to move from the cell interior to the membrane. This action is independent of insulin transport. It is believed that the sulfur atoms of α–Lipoic Acid are responsible for the translocation action. This restoration of normal blood sugar level in turn increases the number of glucose transporters in the membranes of muscle cells. This is a very desirable cycle.

Lipoic Acid supplementation (300 to 600 mg. per day) significantly lowers blood sugar, sorbitol, serum pyruvate and acetoacetate levels while increasing glycogen (stored energy compound for muscles) in muscles and the liver. At the same time, there is an

52

increase in blood sugar utilization by muscle tissues and a reduction in liver glucose output.

Glutathione and Cysteine level increases may play role in normalization of glucose

We know the beneficial effect which lipoic acid has on glutathione and cysteine levels. Both of these amino acids play a critical role in blood sugar regulation.

In Germany where α–Lipoic Acid is currently used as a treatment for diabetic polyneuropathy, researchers made a profound discovery in their efforts to demonstrate the ability of α–Lipoic Acid to enhance glucose utilization. As insulin resistance of skeletal muscle glucose uptake is a prominent feature of Type II diabetes (NIDDM), these interventions to improve insulin sensitivity could be of tremendous benefit.

The study involved 13 patients who received either 1,000 mg. α–Lipoic Acid and the controls who did not. Both groups were comparable in age, body-mass index and duration of diabetes and had a similar degree of insulin resistance at baseline. Administration of α–Lipoic Acid resulted in a significant increase of insulin-stimulated glucose disposal. The metabolic clearance rate for glucose rose by about 50%, whereas the control group did not show any significant change.

This is the first clinical study to show that α–**Lipoic Acid increases insulin stimulated glucose disposal in NIDDM.** The mode of action of α–Lipoic Acid on glucose is not yet completely clear, and its potential use as an antihyperglycemic agent may require further investigation. (Jacob)

CAUTION

Because of the effects of α–Lipoic Acid supplementation to diabetics, individuals may require insulin or oral antidiabetic dose reduction to prevent hypoglycemic states. Close monitoring of blood glucose level is required.

Lipoate Prevents Glucose-induced Protein Modifications

Researchers at the University of California, Berkeley, demonstrated that α–Lipoic Acid prevents the glycation protein damage associated with elevated glucose levels. This study examined the possibility of preventing glycation and subsequent structural modifications of proteins by α–Lipoic Acid as lipoate. Incubation of a protein (bovine serum albumin) at 2 mg./ml. with glucose (500 mg./ml.) in a sterile condition at 37 degrees C for seven days caused glycation and structural damage of the protein structure.

When lipoate (20 mg./ml.) was added, glycation and structural modifications of the protein were significantly prevented. Glycation and inactivation of lysozyme were also prevented by lipoate. The researchers concluded that the results suggested a potential for the therapeutic use of α–Lipoic Acid against diabetes-induced complications. (Suzuki)

Another study at the University of California, Berkeley, to determine the effect of α–Lipoic Acid on protein glycation also showed that this substance may play a role in the prevention of diabetic complications by inhibiting glycation and structural damage of proteins. Bovine serum albumin was incubated with glucose in the presence of α–lipoate or DHLA. Both inhibited bovine serum albumin glycation. (Kawabata)

German researchers have also demonstrated the protective effect of α–Lipoic Acid on membranes with simulation of nondiabetic or diabetic conditions. (Hofmann)

54

α-Lipoic Acid Aids Metabolic Acidosis

The Department of Pediatrics and Child Health, Kurume University, Japan, reported that Lipoic Acid was found beneficial for a patient with defective activity of pyruvate dehydrogenase, 2-oxoglutarate dehydrogenase, and branched-chain keto acid dehydrogenase. This can be a complication associated with diabetes. Ketones are produced in the liver from fats. Excess amounts in the blood can cause serious complications.

Lactic acidosis and accumulation of 3-hydroxybutyrate and other citric acid cycle intermediates were found in an infant with a lethal syndrome of metabolic acidosis and renal tubular acidosis. The activity of the pyruvate dehydrogenase complex, 2-oxoglutarate dehydrogenase, and branched-chain keto acid dehydrogenase were all reduced to between 9 and 29% of control.

In contrast, the activity of lipoamide dehydrogenase was normal. The conversion of leucine and valine to its major metabolic product by fibroblasts derived from the patient was less than 5% of control. Cultivation of the patient's fibroblasts in a medium enriched with α–Lipoic Acid, markedly improved these in vitro conversions of leucine and valine. (Yoshida)

α-Lipoic Acid Improves Nerve Blood Flow, Regenerates Nerves, and Reverses Polyneuropathy

Reduced nerve blood flow due to oxidative stress from elevated glucose levels is a serious problem among diabetics and is so serious that gangrene and amputation of limbs can be the result. α–Lipoic Acid improves nerve blood flow, reduces oxidative stress, and improves distal nerve conduction in diabetic neuropathy. α–Lipoic Acid will reduce oxidative stress in diabetic peripheral nerves and improve neuropathy.

This is reviewed in detail in the following chapter.

Increased Muscle Energy, Decreased Fat Production

A number of research groups have reported how α–Lipoic Acid increases glucose uptake by muscle cells and decreases glucose uptake by fat cells. Dr. M. Khamaisi's group at the University of Negev in Israel reported that the increased glucose transport actually leads to increased energy production. This was confirmed by Dr. Tritschler's group showing increased metabolism and ATP production in muscle tissues, and improved muscle recovery, which permits more work or exercise to be done. The result is more energy production in muscles and less fat stored in the body. This is of interest not only to diabetics, but to us all! (Tritschler)

Neuroprotective Effect of α-Lipoic Acid

Neuropathy (painful swelling and destruction of the nerve and nerve endings) is a problem commonly associated with diabetes due to oxidative stress. Neuropathy can also result from alcoholism*, lead poisoning, or poisoning from certain drugs. Viral infection and autoimmune disorders such as arthritis, lupus erythematosus, and periarteritis can also contribute to neuropathies. In individuals with any of these conditions, higher levels of free radicals accompanied by depressed levels of antioxidants are seen.

Oxidative stress may be greater in neurological tissues because of their constant high rate of oxygen consumption and high mitochondrial density. Mitochondria produce free radicals as "by-products" of normal oxidative metabolic processes which damage mitochondrial DNA, creating a free radical cycle of destruction. This vicious cycle may be largely responsible for neurodegenerative diseases.

Individuals with polyneuropathy hare been found to have lower levels of α–Lipoic Acid. Studies have shown that α–Lipoic Acid and DHLA as potent antioxidants are effective neuroprotective agents.

---

* Excessive alcohol consumption may also cause a Vitamin B-1 (thiamine) deficiency which can also cause nerve damage.

α-Lipoic Acid Protects the Protectors

The generation of radicals is greatly enhanced during postischaemic reoxygenation. (Siesjd, McCord) Our cells are equipped with free radical scavenger enzymes (SOD, peroxidases, catalases) and antioxidants (Vitamins C and E, glutathione) to inactivate them. (Krieglstein) α–Lipoic Acid protects and regenerates these important agents through reduction.

The higher the level of antioxidants present and the longer we can keep these antioxidants regenerating, the longer we are protected from oxidative damage.

α-Lipoic Acid Reverses Nerve Damage

In March 1995, at an international meeting on diabetic neuropathy in Munich, Germany, several researchers reported the results of clinical studies in which α–Lipoic Acid **reversed the damage of diabetes to the nerves, heart and eyes of diabetics.**

Most of the clinical studies were from European universities and clinics. Study after study reported that α–Lipoic Acid safely **regenerated damaged nerves.** The consensus was that α–Lipoic Acid protects through its antioxidant and antiglycemic actions. The conference concluded that α–Lipoic Acid was the agent of choice for the prevention of diabetic complications; neuropathy, cardiomyopathy and retinopathy.

α-Lipoic Acid Improves Neurological Function - Causes Neurite Sprouting

German studies with high doses of α–Lipoic Acid in diabetics have shown that it improves leg nerve conduction velocity as well as heart and gastrointestinal functions. (Reschke)

Dr. D. Ziegler and colleagues at the Heinrich-Heine University in Dusseldorf, Germany, showed that long-term treatment with α–Lipoic Acid induces what is known as nerve "sprouting;" i.e., the growth of new nerve fibers in a regeneration process. In as little as three weeks, there is a significant reduction in pain and numbness. The researchers observed no adverse effects from the high dosage (600 milligrams per day) of α–Lipoic Acid.

Lipoic Acid is believed to cause a dose-dependent sprouting of neurites in nerve cells due to improvement in nerve cell membrane fluidity. In animal experiments, α–Lipoic Acid promoted regeneration after partial denervation. Lipoic Acid improves the blood flow in nerve tissues, improves glucose utilization in the brain and improves basal ganglia function (areas in the cerebrum which are involved in posture and coordination). (Ziegler)

α-Lipoic Acid Reduces Neuropathy

In streptozotocin-induced diabetic neuropathy (SDN), nerve blood flow is reduced by approximately 50%, and oxygen deliverance is greatly reduced. The nerve tissue outside the brain is unique in that compared with nerve tissues inside the brain, glutathione and its related enzymes are reduced to about 10%.

Reperfusion following ischemia will result in reduced protection and a breakdown in the blood-nerve barrier, and an increase in radicals (hydroperoxides). Therefore, the effect to the brain tissue may include swelling and ischemic fiber degeneration.

Laboratory animals experiencing induced diabetic neuropathy (SDN) were evaluated to determine the efficacy of α–Lipoic Acid supplementation in improving nerve blood flow, electrophysiology, and indexes of oxidative stress in peripheral nerves affected by SDN. Nerve blood flow was reduced by 50%. At one month after onset of diabetes and in age-matched controls, α–Lipoic Acid, in doses of 20, 50, and 100 mg./kg, was administered five times per week.

The results were as follows:

♦ α–Lipoic Acid did not affect the nerve blood flow of normal nerves, but improved that of diabetic neuropathy in a dose-dependent manner.

♦ After one month of treatment, α–Lipoic Acid-supplemented rats (100 mg./kg.) exhibited normal nerve blood flow.

♦ The most sensitive and reliable indicator of oxidative stress was a decrease in reduced glutathione, which was significantly lowered in induced diabetic and α–tocopherol-deficient nerves. The levels were improved in a dose-dependent manner in α–Lipoic Acid-supplemented rats.

♦ The conduction velocity of the digital nerve was reduced in diabetic neuropathy and was significantly improved by α–Lipoic Acid, in significant part by reducing the effects of oxidative stress. (Nagamatsu)

NOTE: *A dosage of 100 mg./kg. cannot be used for humans. Rats have a much faster metabolic rate than humans and, because of other differences, we cannot use the same dosage ratio. Most studies show effective dosages for humans closer to 600 mg. total per day.*

The best way to determine the degree of oxidative stress is to look for the degree of reduced glutathione levels, which are significantly reduced in SDN and α–tocopherol deficient nerves. Lipoic Acid

60

treatment resulted in a dose-dependent improvement in individuals with reduced glutathione in SDN, resulting in normal values for the higher doses in α–Lipoic Acid-supplemented rats. The conduction velocity of digital nerve was reduced in SDN and was significantly improved by α–Lipoic Acid. Therefore, these studies suggest that α–Lipoic Acid improves neuropathy, in significant part by reducing the effects of oxidative stress.

Human Studies for Diabetic Peripheral Neuropathy with α–Lipoic Acid

In a 3-week randomized, double-blind placebo-controlled human trial, α–Lipoic Acid was tested on individuals with diabetic neuropathy. The study used 328 Type II diabetic patients with symptomatic peripheral neuropathy who were randomly assigned to treatment with intravenous infusion of α–Lipoic Acid using three different daily doses: 1,200 mg., 600 mg., 100 mg., or a placebo.

Neuropathic symptoms (pain, burning, paraesthesiae, and numbness) were scored at baseline and each visit prior to infusion: 0 (increase in symptoms and pain), 2.5 (no change in symptoms and pain), 5 (significant improvement in symptoms and pain). In addition, a multidimensional specific pain questionnaire (Hamburg Pain Adjective List: HPAL) and the Neuropathy Symptom and Disability Scores were assessed at baseline and day 19*. The total symptoms score decreased from baseline to day 19:

♦ 4.5+3.7 points/ α–Lipoic Acid: 1,200 mg.

♦ 5.0+4.1 points/ α–Lipoic Acid: 600 mg.

♦ 3.3+2.8 points/ α–Lipoic Acid: 100 mg.

♦ 2.6+3.2 points in the placebo

The response rates after 19 days*, defined as an improvement in at least 30%:

♦ 70.8% in α–Lipoic Acid: 1,200 mg.

♦ 82.5% in α–Lipoic Acid: 600 mg.

♦ 65.2% in α–Lipoic Acid: 100 mg.

♦ 57.6% in the placebo

The total HPAL score was significantly reduced in ALA 1,200 mg. and ALA 600 mg. as compared with the placebo after 19 days*.

The rates of adverse events were:

♦ 32.6% in α–Lipoic Acid: 1,200 mg.

♦ 18.2% in α–Lipoic Acid: 600 mg.

♦ 13.6% in α–Lipoic Acid: 100 mg.

♦ 20.7% in the placebo

These findings substantiate that intravenous treatment with α–Lipoic Acid at a dose of 600 mg./day over three weeks is superior to a placebo in reducing symptoms of diabetic peripheral neuropathy without causing significant adverse reactions. Note that there were higher adverse effects in the placebo than the 100 and 600 mg. dosages. (Gries)

Because of the faster metabolic rate of rats, 19 days may not be an accurate estimation of improvement time for humans.

Lipoic Acid and Memory

In mice, α–Lipoic Acid (100 mg./kg. body weight for 15 days) improved performance in an open-field memory test. The α–Lipoic Acid-treated animals performed slightly better than young animals 24 hours after the first test. (Stoll)

Treatment with α–Lipoic Acid did not improve memory in young animals. The authors concluded that α–Lipoic Acid's free radical scavenging ability may improve N-methyl-o-aspartate receptor density, leading to improved memory.

Lipoic Acid Increases Cell Energy Production

Lipoic Acid increased the energy availability in brain and skeletal muscle performance, in a patient with a deficit of mitochondrial function in both brain and muscle.

A woman affected by chronic progressive external ophthalmoplegia and muscle mitochondrial DNA deletion was studied prior to and after one and seven months of treatment with 600 mg. α–Lipoic Acid taken by mouth daily. Before treatment a decreased phosphocreatine content was found in the occipital lobes, accompanied by normal inorganic phosphate level and cytosolic pH. They found a high cytosolic adenosine diphosphate (ADP) concentration and high relative rate of energy metabolism together with a low phosphorylation potential. Muscles showed an abnormal work-energy cost transfer function and a low rate of phosphocreatine recovery during the post-exercise period. All of these findings indicated a deficit of mitochondrial function in both brain and muscle.

Treatment with 600 mg. α–Lipoic Acid daily for 1 month resulted in:

- ◆ **55% increase of brain phosphocreatine,**
- ◆ **72% increase of phosphorylation potential,**
- ◆ **A decrease of calculated ADP and rate of energy metabolism.**

After seven months of treatment, MRS data and mitochondrial function had improved further. Treatment with lipoate also led to a 64% increase in the initial slope of the work-energy cost transfer function in the working calf muscle and worsened the rate of phosphocreatine resynthesis during recovery.

The patient reported subjective improvement of general conditions and muscle performance after therapy. The researchers concluded that the treatment with lipoate caused a relevant increase in levels of energy available in brain and skeletal muscle during exercise. (Barbiroli)

Parkinson's Disease

There is some controversy concerning the potential damage of free radicals catalyzed by monoamine oxidase in **neurodegenerative processes.** There is uncertainty whether products of catecholamine oxidation are relevant factors for neuronal cell death in Parkinson's Disease. To date, products responsible for impairment of biochemical functions essential for cell viability are not yet identified, and the primary site of damage within the cell is unknown. Ammonia, aldehydes and hydrogen peroxide are formed via monoamine oxidase catalyzed oxidations of primary amines. But it is uncertain which of them, if any, is damaging to the cell. (Gotz)

α–Lipoic Acid and The Eye
(Effects on Macular Degeneration and Cataracts)

The eye is highly sensitive to oxidative damage. Laboratory data show that antioxidant vitamins help to protect the retina from oxidative damage initiated in part by absorption of light. The retina distributes α–tocopherol (Vitamin E) in a non-uniform spatial pattern. The region of monkey retinas where carotenoids and Vitamin E are both low corresponds with early signs of age-related macular degeneration (AMD) which often appear in humans. The combination of evidence suggests that carotenoids and antioxidant vitamins may help to retard some of the destructive processes in the retina that lead to age-related degeneration of the macula. The macula is the small oval cone-containing area of the retina near the optic nerve. Accurate sight is dependent upon the focus of the image on the macula.

Research conducted at the Schepens Eye Research Institute, Macular Disease Research Center and other institutions indicates that individuals with low plasma concentrations of carotenoids and antioxidant vitamins and those who smoke cigarettes are at increased risk for AMD. (Snodderly, Seddon)

Researchers at the University of California, Davis, examined 62 elderly rhesus monkeys for the presence and severity of macular drusen. Drusen are

α-LIPOIC ACID EFFECT ON DIABETIC RETINOPATHY

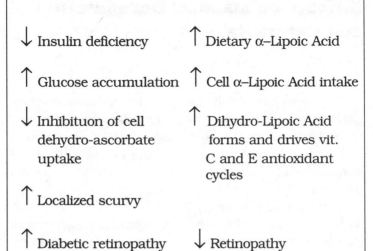

↓ Insulin deficiency   ↑ Dietary α–Lipoic Acid

↑ Glucose accumulation   ↑ Cell α–Lipoic Acid intake

↓ Inhibituon of cell
dehydro-ascorbate
uptake

↑ Dihydro-Lipoic Acid
forms and drives vit.
C and E antioxidant
cycles

↑ Localized scurvy

↑ Diabetic retinopathy   ↓ Retinopathy

Glucose and vitamin C are taken up into cells by the same transport system.

Thiols make low cellular vitamin C work more efficiently.

adapted from Packer, L., "The vitamin E, Ascorbate and Alpha Lipoate Antioxidant Defense System and its Possible Protective Action in Cardiovascular Disease and Diabetes" New Strategies in Prevention and Therapy: The evolution of Antioxidants in Modern Medicine.

identified as yellow spots in the back of the eye indicating degeneration.

Drusen were observed in 47% of the monkeys (which are similar histologically and in clinical appearance to the drusen observed in humans with AMD).

It has been proposed that excessive tissue free radical damage may contribute to the development of AMD. Thus, circulating levels of select components of the free radical defense system and plasma thiobarbituric acid reactive substances (TBARS), an estimate of lipid peroxides, were measured. Monkeys diagnosed with drusen were characterized by alterations in concentrations and activities of several components of the free radical defense system. Alterations were most evident with respect to those enzymes associated with copper.

Excessive oxidative lipid damage may be a factor contributing to the occurrence of macular degeneration. This is demonstrated by the findings of higher plasma TBARS concentrations in animals with greater than 10 drusen compared with animals without drusen. (Olin)

Higher Serum Levels of Antioxidants Reduce Risk of Macular Degeneration

Researchers compared serum levels of carotenoids, Vitamins C and E, and selenium in 421 patients with age-related macular degeneration to 615 controls. Subjects were classified by blood level of the micronutrient (low, medium and high). Persons with carotenoid levels in the medium and high groups, compared with those in the low group, had markedly reduced risks of age-related macular degeneration, with levels of risk reduced to one half and one third, respectively. Although no statistically significant protective effect was found for Vitamin C or E or selenium individually, an antioxidant index that combined all four micronutrient measurements showed statistically significant reductions of risk with increasing levels of the index. Although these results suggest that higher blood levels of micronutrients with antioxidant potential, in particular, carotenoids, may be associated with a decreased risk of the most visually disabling form of age-related macular degeneration.

Tocopherols and Carotenoids in Macular Degeneration

The study group contained a sample of subjects with either retinal pigment abnormalities, the presence of soft drusen, late age-related macular degeneration, or neovascular and exudative macular degeneration. Exudative may refer to hemorrhage (bleeding of the eye) or buildup of serous fluid causing swelling and a multitude of problems.

An equal number of controls were selected from among participants in the Beaver Dam Eye Study. The controls had no evidence of drusen, retinal pigment abnormalities, or late age-related macular degeneration and were matched with cases by age, sex, and current smoking status.

Average levels of individual carotenoids were similar in cases and controls. Average levels of Vitamin E (α–tocopherol) were lower in people with exudative macular degeneration. However, the difference was no longer statistically significant after controlling for levels of cholesterol in the serum.

Persons with low levels of lycopene, the most abundant carotenoid in the blood, were twice as likely to have age-related macular degeneration. Levels of the carotenoids that compose macular pigment (lutein with zeaxanthin) in the serum were unrelated to age-related macular degeneration.

Very low levels of lycopene, but not other dietary carotenoids or tocopherols, were related to age-related macular degeneration. Lower levels of Vitamin E in subjects with exudative macular degeneration, compared with controls, may be explained by lower levels of serum lipids. (Mares-Perlman)

While no studies, to my knowledge, have been done on the regenerative effects of α–Lipoic Acid on carotenoids, it is likely that it would have this effect as it regenerates other antioxidants such as Vitamins E and C, and glutathione.

Cataracts

Cataracts is the term associated with the loss of lens clarity of the eyes reducing one's vision. A gray-white film can be seen behind the pupil. Possible causes of cataracts include:

- Malnutrition
- Amino acid deficiency
- Vitamin deficiency
- Endocrine abnormalities (i.g., diabetes)
- Chemical factors
- Physical factors (i.g., UV radiation)
- Accumulation of toxic products (i.g., cadmium from cigarette smoke)

Several studies indicate high exposure to the sun and radiation are risk factors for cataract development. Of particular risk for the development of cataracts are X rays (gamma rays, beta, UV and IR rays). Low level radiation does not induce cataracts while higher-energy wave or corpuscular radiation does.

Smoking Greatly Increases Cataract Risk

One does not have to be diabetic to suffer from cataracts. One of the major controllable factors contributing to increased risk for cataract formation is smoking. Cigarette smoke contains free radicals and leads to a significant increase in the number of free radicals produced. An abundance of research demonstrates that cigarette smoking increases the risk of developing both nuclear sclerosis and posterior subcapsular cataract. A greater number of cigarettes smoked per day corresponded with a greater degree of severity. (Christen, Klein, Shalini, Ramakrishnan, West)

Smoking Increases Cadmium Level, Reduces Vitamin C, Increases Cataract Risk

Cigarettes also increase the risk of cadmium, heavy metal toxicity.

An estimation of cadmium and Vitamin C levels were performed in the blood and lenses of smokers in three age groups to a maximum age of 58, smoking a minimum of 10 cigarettes a day, compared to non-smokers in the same age groups. The study showed a significant accumulation of cadmium in both the blood and the lenses of the smokers as cadmium seems to have a role in cataractogenesis in smokers. In smokers and non-smokers of two age groups up to a maximum age of 40, both without cataracts, increased levels of cadmium were found in the blood of smokers only, though the extent of accumulation was not as high as in chronic smokers of higher age groups. Vitamin C content of the lens was on the lower side of normal in both chronic smokers in both age groups and non-smokers with nuclear cataract with or without posterior and anterior subcapsular cataract, and there was no significant change brought about by smoking. Vitamin C levels in blood were below normal, in smokers and non-smokers, with and without cataracts. (Ramakrishnan)

These factors have been pointed out due to the specific effects of α–Lipoic Acid regeneration of Vitamin C and also its ability to protect us from cadmium toxicity. (Muller) *See pages 85-86 for more on this subject.*

The Role of Oxidative Processes in Diabetic Retinopathy and Cataract

Several researchers are reporting that the development of the cataract of the eye is an oxidative-degenerative process resembling the physiology of general aging. A measurable parameter is the protein cross-linking or, more generally, the cross-linking and partial loss of function of macromolecules caused by the reaction with aldehydes. A fragment of fatty acid peroxidation is malondialdehyde which is, for example, jointly responsible for the formation of age pigments (lipofuscin) and also for lens opacification. (Kroner)

Two types of oxidative processes are thought to occur in tissues exposed to light: activation of oxygen, and through activated pigment molecules (e.g., flavin-containing substances) which cause the formation of superoxide ($O2$) and singlet oxygen. A defect of the protection or repair capacity of the respective tissue results in the observed irreversible damage by these activated oxygen species.

Lens Damage as an Oxidation Process

At the time of birth, approximately 95% of human lens proteins are water soluble. Disulfide linkages and other covalent bonds (sometimes referred to

71

as cross-linkages) increase with age. The nucleus of the lens assumes an increasingly yellowish color. The oxidation of glycated protein results in the age-dependent accumulation of N-carboxymethyl lysine in the lens. (Dunn) It has been assumed for quite a long time that free radical damage to the amino acids tyrosine and tryptophan (molecules which absorb in the UV range) are responsible for this photodynamic abnormality.

The cornea is affected by "characteristic" aging and by UV light. Degenerative reactions of amino acid (asparagine and glutamine) residues and the degree of hydration of mucopolysaccharides also play a role in lens transparency. (Elstner)

α–Lipoic Acid Prevents Cataracts

Cataract formation is a common diabetic complication. α–Lipoic Acid supplementation decreased cataract formation in a number of trials. In vitro diabetic cataract formation in rat lens cell cultures exposed to high concentrations of glucose was prevented by α–Lipoic Acid. Significant protection of lens ascorbate, tocopherol, and glutathione was also observed in the lipoate-supplemented rats compared to non-supplemented ones. (Kilic)

Researchers at the University of California, Berkeley, including Dr. Packer, investigated the effect of α–Lipoic Acid on cataract formation. They found that in the "cataract-induced" newborn rats, a dose of 25 mg./kg. body weight of α–**Lipoic Acid protected 60% of the animals from cataract formation.**

The "cataract-induced" rats experienced glutathione synthesis inhibition, reduced levels of glutathione, ascorbate and Vitamin E and developed cataracts so this resarch becomes a potential model for studying the role of therapeutic antioxidants in protecting animals from cataract formation.

The major biochemical changes in the lens associated with the protective effect of α–Lipoic Acid were:

♦ Increased glutathione
♦ Increased ascorbate
♦ Increased Vitamin E levels

Treatment with α–Lipoic Acid also restored the protective activities of glutathione peroxidase, catalase, and ascorbate free radical reductase in lenses of the treated animals.

The researchers concluded that α–Lipoic Acid may take over some of the functions of glutathione (e.g., maintaining the higher level of ascorbate, indirect participation in Vitamin E recycling). The increase of glutathione level in lens tissue caused by lipoate could be due also to a direct protection of protein thiols. Thus, α–Lipoic Acid could be of potential therapeutic use in preventing cataracts and their complications. (Maitra)

Dr. Packer hypothesizes that α–Lipoic Acid prevents oxidative stress in diabetic conditions by sparing Vitamin C. Since Vitamin C and glucose share the same carrier in non-insulin-dependent tissues, the elevated blood glucose in diabetes competitively inhibits the cell entry of Vitamin C, resulting in localized intracellular Vitamin C deficiency.

Supplemented α–Lipoic Acid utilizes other transport systems to enter the cells, is converted to DHLA, and recycles Vitamin C. This would explain its protective effect in diabetic cataractogenesis, as well as many other complications of diabetes.

R-Lipoic Acid More Effective Than S-Lipoic Acid Against Cataracts

The effect of α–Lipoic Acid was tested on the formation of opacity in normal rat lenses incubated with glucose as a model for in-vivo diabetic cataractogenesis. Control lenses, incubated with glucose, did not develop opacities. Formation of lens opacities in vitro was correlated with lactate dehydrogenase (LDH) leakage into the incubation medium which is an indication of loss of cell integrity. Opacity formation and lactate dehydrogenase leakage, resulting from incubation in glucose, were both suppressed by the addition of racemic α–Lipoic Acid (R-α–Lipoic Acid).

Addition of racemic α–Lipoic Acid **reduced the damaging effects to the lens by one-half,** while S-α–Lipoic Acid showed no benefit. This is consistent with the hypothesis that R-lipoic is the more active form. (Trevithick)

α–Lipoic Acid and HIV

Acquired immunodeficiency syndrome (AIDS) results from infection with a human immunodeficiency virus (HIV). The virus destroys T-cells, white blood cells which play a key role in the immune system which protects us from illness. Compromised immunity makes one more susceptible to illness from a multitude of invasions ranging from candida albicans to cancer.

A number of beneficial effects have been noted through supplementation of α–Lipoic Acid, some of these through its direct antioxidant effects against replication of the virus, but also indirectly through beneficial effects on white blood cells, including T-cells. It is assumed that the higher the viral load in the body, the more difficult it is to maintain T-cells and a necessary degree of immunity.

Antioxidants Enhance Immune Response

Dietary deficiencies of antioxidants can depress immune function through a variety of ways. Free radicals can inactivate white blood cells such as neutrophils and macrophages, and other protective agents such as trypsin (causing inflammatory damage).

Studies show immune enhancement with supplementation of Vitamin E and other antioxidants. Higher intakes of antioxidants are associated with lower rates of infection and higher levels of antibodies.

HIV-infected patients are reported to be deficient in various antioxidants. (Bendich, Buhl, Dworkin, Bohl)

German researchers investigated the effects of α–Lipoic Acid supplementation (150 mg. three times daily) in 12 HIV-positive individuals. After 14 days, the following results were noted:

♦ **Plasma ascorbate and glutathione increased**

♦ **Markers of plasma lipid peroxidation decreased**

♦ **T-helper cells increased in six patients**

♦ **The T-helper: T suppressor cell ratio improved in six patients (Fuchs)**

Also, in cultured cells, α–Lipoic Acid and Dihydrolipoic Acid prevented HIV replication and the activation of NF-kappa B transcription factor, which is regulated by oxidative stress.

Lipoic Acid Blocks Replication of HIV-1 and other Viruses

HIV replication is activated by release and binding of nuclear factor-kappa B (NF-kappa B) on the binding sights on the genetic material (DNA) of the virus. When NF-kappa B is activated (through oxidation), it binds to the binding sites on the DNA setting the replication processes in motion.

Remember though, NF-kappa B also regulates a wide variety of cellular and viral genes in addition to HIV. Therefore, oxidative stress plays a role in several additional aspects of HIV infection. (Legrand-Poels) Oxidative stress is also involved in immunosuppression (Freed, Aune), and tumor initiation and promotion. (Cerutti)

Researchers at the University of California, Berkeley, have also demonstrated the potential for α–Lipoic Acid to block replication of HIV and other viruses. They demonstrated that α–lipoate/DHLA influences the DNA binding activity of NF-kappa B. (Suzuki)

According to Dr. Packer, human studies at the University of California, Berkeley, with α–lipoate are in the planning stages for the near future.

α–**Lipoic Acid Blocks Activation of HIV**

Additional studies have confirmed reports that α–Lipoic Acid can block the activation of NF-kappa B and subsequently HIV transcription, and can be used as therapeutic agents for AIDS.

Incubation of T-cells with α–Lipoic Acid, prior to the stimulation of cells, was found to inhibit NF-kappa B activation. The inhibitory action of α–Lipoic Acid was found to be very potent as only a small amount (4 mM) was needed for a complete inhibition, compared to the 20 mM required for N-acetylcysteine (NAC). The results indicated that α–Lipoic Acid may be effective in AIDS therapeutics. (Suzuki)

Lipoic Acid: Glutathione in T-cells

Supplemental α–Lipoic Acid causes a rapid increase of intracellular unbound thiols in Jurkat cells, a human T-lymphocyte cell line. The rise of cellular thiols is a result of the cellular uptake and reduction of α–Lipoic Acid to DHLA and a rise in intracellular glutathione. Although the level of DHLA is 40 fold lower than glutathione, the cellular concentration of DHLA might be responsible for the modulation of total cellular thiol levels. Rises in glutathione correlate with the levels of intracellular DHLA.

Lipoic Acid had no effect on glutathione levels when cells were grown in a cysteine-free medium (an essential amino acid for glutathione synthesis) or after administration of an inhibitor of cysteine synthetase. The rise in glutathione was still observed after the administration of a protein synthesis inhibitor.

Because of the ability of α–Lipoic Acid to modulate glutathione levels in low dosages, the researchers recommended that α–Lipoic Acid administration should be considered as a potential therapeutic agent in oxidative stress diseases with glutathione abnormalities, including HIV infection. (Han, Derick & Packer)

Japanese researchers have also demonstrated inhibitory effects of α–Lipoic Acid against HIV replication showing that α–**Lipoic Acid and N-acetycysteine (NAC) significantly depressed HIV-1 reproduction activity.** (Shoji)

Implications of Effect on Viral Load

It is assumed that one's viral load level may provide an indicatation of health status as the range of health varies so greatly among individuals who are HIV-positive. Some individuals carry the virus for 10 years before any serious health problems develop. In others, symptoms present themselves a short time after assumed infection. Does this reflect one's general state of health and the body's ability to slow replication of the virus?

If α–Lipoic Acid supplementation can reduce one's viral load, or slow its replication in the body, the potential benefit could be tremendous indeed. But without research dollars to support large-scale investigations, like many other "natural" unpatentable substances, we may have to "wait and see" what the actual impact will be. This is not an AIDS cure, but it could be a needed support nutrient for immune enhancement for prolonged and improved quality of life.

α-Lipoic Acid and Heart Disease/LDL Cholesterol

Oxidation of low density lipoprotein (LDL) plays a key role in the pathogenesis of atherosclerosis. Many studies suggest that antioxidants may protect LDL against oxidation. As previously indicated, α–Lipoic Acid recycles Vitamins C and E and is synergistic with these antioxidants in warding off free radical damage.

Blood samples of 36 African Americans, ages 16 to 37, showed an inverse correlation between LDL α–tocopherol content and LDL oxidation rate. LDL samples with **higher α–tocopherol content exhibit slower LDL oxidation lag rates,** demonstrating the ability of Vitamin E to increase LDL resistance to oxidation. (Zhang)

Oxidative Stress Decreased In Coronary Heart Disease Patients with Antioxidant

Antioxidant levels of β-carotene and ascorbic acid in blood plasma remain consistent with age, whereas α–tocopherol levels increase from age 20 up to 59 years, and decrease in individuals older than age 60. Coronary heart disease patients show decreased plasma levels of α–tocopherol accompanied by increased activity of erythrocyte SOD, glutathione peroxidase, and catalase. (Junqueira)

α -Lipoic Acid Inhibits Lipid Peroxidation

Studies show that α–Lipoic Acid is effective in the protection of the liver, brain, skin, and heart tissues against lipid peroxidation. Following two weeks of supplementation, the most dramatic responses were shown in the liver, but the brain and skin respond readily. The heart tissues were slow to respond. (Serbinova)

The effects are due largely to the recycling effect that α–Lipoic Acid has on the natural antioxidants such as Vitamin E, ubiquinols and the carotenoids, the major antioxidants that protect the fat-soluble areas such as cell membranes from damage.

α -Lipoic Acid Protects Apolproteins of Human LDL Against Oxidative Damage

Lipoic Acid is a coenzyme for the pyruvate dehydrogenase complex in the mitochondrial matrix. Reactive oxygen species are implicated in most, if not all, human diseases. Upon stimulation, neutrophils produce oxygen radicals, superoxide and hydrogen peroxide. Neutrophils also release enzymes which convert chloride to the very powerful oxidant hypochlorous acid (HOCL). These contribute to the bactericidal action of neutrophils. However, the damaging effect of these products is not limited to bacteria; the surrounding tissue is also vulnerable.

Studies on LDL oxidative modification by hypochlorous acid have been reported. The HOCL induced damage is limited to the protein portion of

80

the molecule. Another research team led by Dr. Packer presented the ability of lipoate to protect apolproteinB against oxidative modification by HOCL. They demonstrated that with increased α–Lipoic Acid antioxidant concentrations, apolproteinB carbonyls were decreased, and the loss of apolproteinB free-SH groups was inhibited. Furthermore, the results demonstrated that in this case, dihydrolipoic Acid is even more efficient than α–Lipoic Acid in protection against hypochlorite-mediated apolproteinB oxidative damage. (Yan & Packer)

α -Lipoic Acid Prevents Glycation of Hemoglobin and Prevents Iron Oxidation

Hemoglobin is a blood constituent consisting of protein and iron. It is responsible for the transport of oxygen throughout the body. Like all tissues in the body, it is susceptible to oxidative damage. If iron is oxidized, a highly potent radical is produced and circulates in the vulnerable arteries of the body which bring blood and oxygen to all vital organs. α–Lipoic Acid prevents this oxidation from occurring. (Novak)

α -Lipoic Acid Speeds Recovery Following Heart Attack and Stroke - Prevents Free Radical Damage

When there is an interruption in blood flow or oxygen supply to a tissue, it is called ischemia. Examples would be a heart attack or stroke where the blood supply becomes blocked to the heart or the brain. Reperfusion is the term associated with the administration of drugs which will restore blood flow. When this happens, reperfusion injury occurs as a

81

burst of free radicals is produced during reoxygenation of that tissue. It is important in cardiac tissue (as in the introduction of clot-dissolving drugs for the treatment of heart attack) and in the brain.

Agents that prevent ischemia-reperfusion injury may therefore prove important during open-heart surgery, and in the treatment of stroke and other conditions that cause interruption of blood flow.

Dr. Packer demonstrated that α–Lipoic Acid prevented damage following 40 minutes of ischemia and 20 minutes of reperfusion. The mechanical recovery of hearts from the Lipoic Acid-supplemented group was 68% as compared to 34% recovery of the hearts obtained from rats fed the normal diet. (Packer)

The content of end products of lipid peroxidation (fluorescence products) after 60 minutes of perfusion was approximately doubled both in the hearts obtained from control animals and in animals given α–Lipoic Acid. When hearts were subjected to 40 minutes of ischemia and 20 minutes of reperfusion, fluorescent products increased five-fold. α-Lipoic Acid prevented the accumulation of lipid peroxidation products. In this group the content of fluorescence products increased only 2.8 times.

The protective effects of DHLA against rat myocardial ischemia-reperfusion injury are dependent on Vitamin E, suggesting that α–Lipoic Acid functions in this system by regenerating tocopherol and decreasing damage caused by free radicals. (Haramaki, Serbinova)

Assadnazari reported that DHLA added to the reperfusion buffer accelerating the recovery of aortic flow during reperfusion. DHLA also appeared to increase ATP synthesis (energy) in the heart. (Assadnazari)

82

α-Lipoic Acid Protects Internal Organs

Lipoic Acid is presently used in therapy for a variety of liver and kidney disorders. Free radical formation as a part of normal metabolism occurs throughout the body in every organ and gland.

α-Lipoic Acid Reduces Kidney Oxidative Stress

Kidney damage may be due to sugar damage to protein tissues (glycation). This is a common complication of diabetes. Kidney disease is responsible for only 10% of all deaths, but for 50 to 60% of deaths of insulin-dependent diabetics.

The cause of diabetic kidney disease is not completely understood. It is due in part to high amounts of protein breakdown products (proteinuria). Without insulin production, the production of catabolic hormones increases. The overproduction of these hormones causes harmful effects to important proteins and fatty acids in the body. Further, this can contribute to ketoacidosis (excess production of ketone bodies (such as acetone) due to the breakdown of proteins. Excess ketone bodies can overwhelm the system causing depletion of cations such as sodium. This puts tremendous stress on the kidneys, and the pH of the blood can drop to dangerous levels.

Kidney stress also comes from elevated glucose. When blood glucose levels exceed the "renal threshold" (160-200 mg./dl.), additional glucose cannot be reabsorbed and the glucose is excreted in the urine. This also draws water from the cells which can cause dehydration (thirst, dry skin, etc.).

To examine the protective effects of α–Lipoic Acid on the kidneys, researchers artificially induced a higher oxidation level and examined the effects of α–Lipoic Acid administration. They first administered an agent (sodium glyoxylate) which increased liver glycollate oxidase radical formation (the major enzyme encouraging free radical formation). This significantly raised the levels of renal tissue calcium and oxalate (reflected simultaneously in their urinary levels). α–Lipoic Acid administration had the following effects:

- ◆ **Lowered** oxalate levels in the kidney and urine.
- ◆ **Decreased** glycollate oxidase activity.

The researchers concluded that the possibility of regulating oxalate metabolism with the use of α–Lipoic Acid by way of inhibiting liver glycollate oxidase looks promising. (Jayanthi)

α-**Lipoic Acid Prevents Kidney Stones**

α–Lipoic Acid has demonstrated the ability to prevent kidney stone formation (calculogenosis) in laboratory animals. Kidney stones are formed from mineral salts and can cause irritation, organ obstruction and great pain. Increased tissue cholesterol and triglycerides and low phospholipid levels are suggested as risk factors for the development of stones.

The effects of α–Lipoic Acid on altered tissue

84

lipid levels were examined during experimental kidney stone formation. **Lipoic Acid treatment reduced tissue cholesterol and triglyceride levels significantly and raised phospholipids.** These alterations were suspected to play a role in the reduced stone formation. (Jayanthi, 1992)

In another study, the effects of α–Lipoic Acid were studied on certain key carbohydrate metabolizing enzymes in the tissues of calculogenic rats. **The two major enzymes, glucose-6-phosphatase (G6P) and fructose-1-6 diphosphatase (FDP) were significantly inhibited in tissues of calculogenic rats. Lipoic Acid also reduced the enzyme activities significantly.** The citric acid cycle enzymes were not influenced appreciably. The observed alterations are likely to be due to the regulatory effects of oxalate and lipoate on the enzyme systems. (Jayanthi)

α-Lipoic Acid Protects Us From Cigarette Smoke

Cigarette smoke contains a number of free radical species. Since many of the diseases caused by smoking involve, at least in part, free radical-mediated processes, it has been proposed that the free radicals in cigarette smoke contribute to smoking-related diseases.

The effects of cigarette smoke on lung fluids have been investigated using plasma as a model system. Supplemental DHLA is protective against cigarette smoke-induced oxidation of antioxidants, proteins, and lipids. (Cross)

DHLA also partially protects leukocytes from the damaging effects of cigarette smoke. (Tsuchiya) This effect may be due to scavenging of oxidants in the aqueous or lipid phases, or to regeneration of ascorbic acid that has been converted to ascorbyl radical as

85

it is oxidized by cigarette smoke components. In this regard, DHLA could play a role in minimizing the pathological consequences of smoking.

Lipoic Acid As Metal-Chelating Antioxidant

Heavy metals such as iron, copper, lead, mercury, arsenide, and cadmium can be very damaging in the body. Among other problems they can serve as catalysts for the formation of free radicals in the cells.

α–Lipoic Acid as a therapeutic metal-chelating antioxidant make it a good candidate for the treatment of heavy metal poisoning. It may be especially effective against arsenide, cadmium, and mercury. α–Lipoic Acid administration greatly increases the rate of elimination of heavy metals. (Grune)

α–Lipoic Acid has a profound dose-dependent inhibitory effect upon copper-catalyzed ascorbic acid oxidation and also copper catalyzed liposomal peroxidation. α–Lipoic Acid also inhibited intracellular free radical production of H_2O_2 in erythrocytes challenged with ascorbate, a process thought to be mediated by copper within the erythrocyte. (Tritschler)

Exposure of isolated hepatocytes to α–Lipoic Acid or DHLA resulted in reduced cadmium-induced membrane damage, reduced peroxidation, and the reduced depletion of cellular glutathione. These findings were extended to a rat model in which 30 mg. α–Lipoic Acid completely prevented cadmium-induced peroxidation in the brain, heart and testes. (Sumathi)

Lipoic Acid Protects Liver from Cadmium Toxicity

Acute cadmium toxicity causes severe liver disturbances. Isolated rat liver cells were coincubated

86

with lipoate or DHLA for up to 90 minutes. Following exposure to cadmium, uptake was deminished with both lipoate and DHLA in correspondence to time and concentration. Cadmium-induced damage was decreased as cadmium-stimulated lipid peroxidation decreased.

Lipoate was not as effective as DHLA as a protectant. Lipoate increased extracellular acid-soluble thiols different from glutathione. It is suggested that DHLA primarily protects cells by extracellular chelation of cadmium, whereas intracellular reduction of lipoate to the DHLA provides both intra- and extracellular cadmium chelation/protection. (Muller)

Mushroom Poisoning -- Elimination of Toxins

Historically, mortality after Amanita mushroom ingestion has ranged from 50% to 90%. Prompt and aggressive therapeutic measures must be instituted quickly to improve the outcome. Successful treatment has been reported using combined therapy of α–Lipoic Acid and hemoperfusion. (Piering)

Over a period of 15 years, 41 patients with Amanita mushroom poisoning were treated at the University Hospital of Lund, Sweden, where α–Lipoic Acid is used in conjunction with other substances for treatment. Treatment consisted of fluid and electrolyte replacement; oral activated charcoal and lactulose; i.v. penicillin, α–Lipoic Acid, and silibinin; combined hemodialysis and hemoperfusion in two 8 hour sessions; and a special diet.

The combination of treatment modalities accelerated the elimination of amatoxin from the patients' bodies. The longest period of hospitalization, about 13 days, was required by Group C.

All patients improved and were discharged from

the hospital without symptoms. No difficulties were later reported for the majority of those moderately and severely poisoned. The researchers concluded that intensive combined treatment applied in these cases is effective in relieving patients with both moderate and severe amanitin poisoning. (Sabeel)

According to some experts such as Dr. Packer, while Lipoic Acid is often used for therapy in conditions that involve liver pathology, especially mushroom poisoning and alcoholic liver degeneration, there is little evidence that α–Lipoic Acid is useful in either of these conditions.

Although case reports describe complete recovery from mushroom (Amanita) poisoning in patients treated with α–Lipoic Acid, 10 to 50% of victims recover without α–Lipoic Acid treatment. (Packer)

Protection from Effects of Alcohol

Several in vitro studies have indicated that α–Lipoic Acid supplementation might be beneficial in alcoholic liver disease. (Wickramasing) However, some researchers feel that these studies suffered from lack of control groups, lack of statistical analysis or comparative treatments with α–Lipoic Acid. In one controlled, double-blind, long-term study, α–Lipoic Acid had no effect on the course of alcohol-related liver disease. (Marshall) Therefore, its use for the treatment of alcoholic liver disease is not recommended. (Packer)

However, it should be pointed out that due to the beneficial effects of α–Lipoic Acid on glutathione and cysteine levels and the protective effects against neuropathy, further research may be warranted for α–Lipoic Acid as a conjunctive treatment.

α-Lipoic Acid as a Nutritional Supplement

Lipoic Acid has been safely used therapeutically to treat diabetic neuropathy for over 30 years at dosages from 300 to 600 mg. daily. Even at this high dose, there have been no serious adverse effects reported. No studies indicate any carcinogenic or teratogenic (birth defect causing) effects.

Lipoic Acid is absorbed from the diet, transported to the tissues and taken up by cells where a majority is rapidly converted to DHLA. Studies show that α–Lipoic Acid protects us against deficiencies of Vitamins E and C.

Dosage

Supplementation for healthy individuals is usually between 20 and 50 mg. daily.

Therapeutic dosages greatly depend on the intent of benefit and severity of one's health situation. As always when a medical problem exists, a doctor's guidance should be sought before taking any supplement. Because of the improved glucose utilization for diabetics, individuals should monitor blood sugar levels closely to determine possible appropriate modifications in their regimen.

Studies have demonstrated that optimal results for diabetics are achieved with about 600 mg. daily

(200 mg. taken 3 times daily). Better results were not necessarily seen at dosages above 1,000 mg. daily, so therefore are not recommended.

Lethal dosage (LD_{50}) is approximately 400 to 500 mg./kg. after oral dosing in dogs. (Packer) There are 2.2 lbs. in 1 kilogram. Therefore, lethal dosage for a 150 pound human is around 34,000 mg. daily (i.e., 34 grams, or 681 50 mg. capsules). But, if you were to take over 600 capsules of just about anything, it would probably kill you. α–Lipoic Acid is extremely safe.

Side Effects

In humans, the only adverse effects reported to date are possible allergic skin reaction (which is a risk for essentially all foods) and hypoglycemia in diabetics as a consequence of improved glucose utilization with very high doses. (Asta-Medica)

As α-Lipoic Acid is a sulphur-bearing compound, there is a potential risk of adverse effects upon the gastrointestinal tract, and some people using high dosages may experience gas, distension or a bloated feeling.

Availability

α -Lipoic Acid is currently manufactured by only a few companies in Russia, Japan, Italy and China. It can be purchased in many local pharmacies and health food stores. Many physicians are also aware of the benefits of Lipoic Acid and provide it for their patients. If you feel that you can benefit from α-Lipoic Acid but your physician is not familiar with its use for your medical situation, give him or her a copy of this book.

At this writing, therapeutic dosages (600 mg./day) are rather expensive for the average person

- $70 to $80 a month - and as a nutritional supplement, it is not covered by most health plans.

Hopefully, as more people learn about the benefits, the demand will increase, bringing down the cost.

Questions and Answers:

Q: If α-Lipoic Acid is called the potato antioxidant, can't we get the benefits by eating a lot of potatoes?

A: α-Lipoic Acid is found in potatoes and other foods as as carrots, yams, sweet potatoes, beets, and also red meat, but the amount is so little that supplementation is required in order for us to obtain any antioxidant protection.

α-Lipoic Acid is sometimes called the potato antioxidant because in the 1930's it was discovered that a so-called "potato growth factor," was necessary for growth of certain bacteria. In 1957, the compound was extracted and identified as α-Lipoic Acid.

Q: Because α–Lipoic Acid regenerates other antioxidants in the body such as glutathione and Vitamins C and E, does this mean we no longer need to supplement these?

A: Studies show that many of these antioxidants actually have a synergistic effect on each other when taken together. Hence, they work better taken together than taken separately.

Q: What is the best way to take α–Lipoic Acid?

A: Because most antioxidants are water-soluble and need to be taken 2 to 3 times a day, and because we know of the synergistic action when taken together, it is best to take it with your other antioxidants.

According to Dr. Packer, "the half life of α–Lipoic Acid in the blood is relatively short, 6 to 8 hours, but I would expect that its life in the tissue would be longer. We have seen some confirmation of this invitro."

Q: What will I feel after taking α-Lipoic Acid?

A: This greatly depends on the individual situation of each person, their health status and the dosage they are using.

In most cases, because it works on a cellular level, you won't really feel anything. Some individuals may feel as if they have more energy generally.

Individuals with health problems such as diabetes may experience improvements after a few weeks in various areas. Some reports indicate that glucose regulation and neuropathy may improve after just 30 days.

Q: Are there any long-term side effects of taking α-Lipoic Acid?

A: Taken in the daily dosage range of 20 to 200 mg. for average individuals and up to 1,200 mg. in individuals with degenerative health problems such as arthritis, lupus, diabetes, HIV, etc., studies do not indicate that side effects are likely. α–Lipoic Acid is produced in the body. If you think about it, it seems there would be more adverse effects to **not** taking it.

I spoke to Dr. Packer about the side effects of α–Lipoic Acid. He reported that he was not aware of any serious side effects reported at 600 mg. taken orally. He pointed out, however, that any substance used to extreme levels can be dangerous. The toxic dosage is a very high amount (50 or 60 grams) so lipoic acid seems to be very safe.

I also asked Dr. Packer about the potential proxidant effects if taken in excess. He agreed that antioxidants can turn into proxidants and create free radicals.

For example, UVAB exposure causes Vitamin E in the skin to oxidate. But if there is enough Vitamin C present to quench the free radicals, it all balances out.

He pointed out that there are companies that do tests which measure one's levels of antioxidants, something one may consider to obtain balance.

Dr. Packer reported that he himself supplements α–Lipoic Acid, but wouldn't say how much because everyone is different and requires different amounts.

Q: Some of the effects of α-Lipoic Acid seem too good to be true, such as its ability to actually reverse neuropathy? I thought nerve cells and brain cells could not be restored after they die?

A: All cells in the body will renew themselves over and over until the cell becomes damaged and dies. In many cases, new cells form and take their places. This is more evident in areas where cells grow rapidly such as the skin, compared to slow growing areas (nerve and brain cells, liver cells, bone cells, etc.)

In the case of diabetic neuropathy, where glycation destroys nerve endings, α–Lipoic Acid can help prevent further damage from occurring and allow the normal regenerative processes of the body to take place. It is not completely clear how α–Lipoic Acid promotes neurite sprouting, or reduce pain, burning and numbness. Because no other substance has shown such potential these effects on neuropathy are very encouraging for those suffering individuals.

Q: If it is so great, why hasn't my doctor heard about α-Lipoic Acid?

A: α–Lipoic Acid is a nutritional substance as it is naturally found in food and the body (and therefore cannot be patented). Unfortunately, many doctors do not take the time or have the time to educate themselves on the many nutritional substances available to us for our benefit.

As a nutritional found in nature and manufactured by the body, α-Lipoic Acid cannot be patented, meaning anyone can manufacture and sell it. For this reason, US pharmaceutical companies are not going to invest a great deal of money to educate either physicians or the public. When a new drug is released, pharmaceutical companies spend hundreds of thousands of advertising dollars in magazines (often two and three pages), television and radio, offer free medical seminars for doctors and pharmacists, plus provide doctors with free samples to entice us to try their new product. They can do this because if we like it, we have to buy it from them. It is patent protected and no one else has it. ABC Company is not going to spend $500,000.00 in advertising and education if the consumer can buy the same thing from Company X.

It therefore is the responsibility of each person to learn about the substances that will most benefit him or her. Nutritional science is becoming more and more complicated. We now need to learn about what the body needs to maintain proper balance with a variety of complex nutritionals like DHEA (dehydroepiandrosterone), MCHC (microcrystalline hydroxyapatite), NADH, and α-Lipoic Acid!

We cannot rely upon our physician to always

know what is best for us. If you are so fortunate to have a doctor who does care enough to do this research for you and his other patients, you should be very grateful. They are hard to come by.

Q: If the "r" form of α-Lipoic Acid works more effectively that the "s", shouldn't we look for the "r" form in a supplement instead of the "s"?

A: One or more studies have so far indicated that r-α-Lipoic Acid may be more effective that s-α-Lipoic Acid to prevent cataracts, but it does not necessarily mean that r-α-Lipoic Acid is more effective overall. We really don't have enough information to make that determination.

It seems that most commercial α–Lipoic Acid available is a mix containing both r-α-Lipoic Acid and s-α-Lipoic Acid.

Q: Could you explain the effects of ALA with regard to HIV?

A: There are two activation sights located on the genetic material of the virus which regulate replication of the cell. These are known as NF-kappa B binding sites. NF-kappa B is not just involved in HIV replication; it also regulates replication of other viruses and also inflammation throughout the body and a wide variety of additional cellular responses. Therefore, this is of importance to individuals with arthritis and other inflammatory conditions.

Oxidative stress is known to activate the transcription initiating either replication of the virus or inflammation, etc. Oxidative stress seems to have a negative effect on the immune system as a whole. As α–Lipoic Acid has shown to reduce oxidative stress in the body, this is of great benefit.

There are also studies showing the positive

effect of α–Lipoic Acid supplementation on levels of glutathione and cysteine for HIV individuals.

Dr. Packer informed me that researchers at the University of California, Berkeley, are planning to further investigate the effects of lipoate on individuals with HIV in the very near future.

Q: Will ALA benefit only individuals who have depressed levels?

A: Not necessarily. In many cases it depends on the degree of oxidative stress in the body. The key is to obtain balance between antioxidants and free radicals in the body.

In some situations, α-Lipoic Acid has shown to have effects only in individuals who had depressed levels, such as diabetics in regards to glucose regulation. For the most part, the majority of individuals can benefit from the added antioxidant protection offered by α–Lipoic Acid.

Bibliography

Achmad, T.H., Rao, G.S., Chemotaxis of human blood monocytes toward endothelin-1 and the influence of calcium channel blockers. Institute of Clinical Biochemistry, University of Bonn, Germany. Biochem Biophys Res Commun 1992 Dec 15;189(2):994-1000.

Ahmad, T., Frischer, H.J., Lab Clin Med 1985 Apr;105(4):464-71.

Altenkirch, H., Stoltenburg-Didinger, G., Wagner, H.M., Herrmann, J., and Walter, G., Neuroltoxicoll. Teratol 12 (1990):619-622.

Amatuni, V.G.; Malaian, K.L.; Zakaharian, A.K., "The effect of a single dose of nifedipine, intal, sodium thiosulfate and Essentiale on the blood level of calcium, hydroperoxides, thiol compounds and prostaglandins in bronchial asthma patients] Ter Arkh 1992;64(3):61-4.

Antioxidant status and neovascular age-related macular degeneration. Eye Disease Case-Control Study Group [published errata appear in Arch Ophthalmol 1993 Sep;111(9):1228, 1993 Oct;111(10):1366 and 1993 Nov;111(11):1499] Arch Ophthalmol 1993 Jan;111(1):104-9.

AstaMedica, α–Lipoic Acid prescribing information, Asta Medica AG, Frankfurt, Germany.

Aune. T.M., Pierce, C.W. Conversion of soluble immune response suppressor to macrophage-derived suppressor factor by peroxide Proc. National Academy of Sciences USA (1981) 78: 5099-5103.

Azzadnazari, H., Simmer, G., Freisleben, H.J., et al Cardioprotective efficiency of dihydroα–Lipoic Acid in working rat hearts during hypoxia and reoxygenation Arnzmeimittel-Forsch (1993) 43: 425-432.

Azzini, M.; Girelli, D.; Olivieri, O.; Guarini, P.; Stanzial, AM.; Frigo, A.; Milanino, R.; et al Fatty acids and antioxidant micronutrients in psoriatic arthritis. Institute of Medical Pathology, University of Verona, Italy. J Rheumatol 1995 Jan;22(1):103-8.

Backman-Gullers, B., Hannestad, U., Nilsson, L., Sorbo, B., Studies on lipoamidase: characterization of the enzyme in human serum and breast milk. Department of Clinical Chemistry, Faculty of Health Sciences, Linkoping University, Sweden. Clin Chim Acta 1990 Oct 31;191(1-2):49-60.

Baker, J.C., Andrews, P.C., Roche Recombinant expression and evaluation of the lipoyl domains of the dihydrolipoyl acetyltransferase component of the human pyruvate dehydrogenase complex. Arch Biochem Biophys 1995 Feb 1;316(2):926-40.

Barber, D.A., Harris, S.R., Oxygen free radicals and antioxidants: a review. Department of Surgery, Mayo Clinic & Foundation, Rochester, Minn. Am Pharm 1994 Sep;NS34(9):26-35.

Barbiroli, B., Medori, R., Tritschler, H.J., Klopstock, T., Seibel, P., Reichmann, H., Iotti, S., Lodi, R., Zaniol, P., Lipoic (thioctic) acid increases brain energy availability and skeletal muscle performance as shown by in vivo 31P-MRS in a patient with mitochondrial cytopathy. J Neurol 1995 Jul;242(7):472-7.

Bendich, Adrianne, " Antioxidant Micronutrients Annals of the New York Academy of Sciences,Vol 587, 1990. 168-180.

Bolevic, S., Kogan, Daniyak The Antioxidant Effect of Platelets in the Norm and Correction of its Disturbance in Asthmatic Patients, Sechenov Moscow Medical Academy, Russia *Oxidants and Antioxidants in Biology*, Oxygen Club of California, Annual Meeting, March 1995.

Bolevic, S., Kogan, S. ,Grachev, Geppe, Dairova & Dinilyak. CO2 Antioxidant Effect on the Development of Asthma. Sechenov Moscow Medical Academy, Moscow, Russia *Oxidants and Antioxidants in Biology*, Oxygen Club of California, Annual Meeting, March 1995.

Boljevic, S., Daniljak, I.G., Kogan, A.H., "Changes in free radicals and possibility of their correction in patients with bronchial asthma Katedra za unutrasnje bolesti br. 2, Prvog medicinskog fakulteta, Moskovske medicinske akademije I. M. Secenov. Vojnosanit Pregl 1993 Jan-Feb;50(1):3-18.

Buhl, R., Jaffe. H.A.. et. al., Glutathione deficiency and HIV. Lancet, (1990) 335: 546.

Busse, E., Zimmer., G., Schopohl, B., Kornhuber, B., Influence of α–Lipoic Acid on intracellular glutathione in vitro and in vivo. Abteilung fur Hamatologie und Onkologie, Johann Wolfgang Goethe-Universitat, Frankfurt/Main Fed. Rep. of Germany. Arzneimittelforschung 1992 Jun;42(6):829-31.

Byrd, D.J., Krohn, H.P., Winkler, L., Steinborn, C., Hadam, M., Brodehl, J., Neonatal pyruvate dehydrogenase deficiency with lipoate responsive lactic acidaemia and hyperammonaemia. Eur J Pediatr 1989 Apr;148(6):543-7.

Chen, C., Loo, G.. Inhibition of lecithin: cholesterol acyltransferase activity in human blood plasma by cigarette smoke extract and reactivealdehydes. J Biochem Toxicol 1995 Jun;10(3):121-8

Christen, W.G,. Manson, J.E., Seddon, J.M,. Glynn, R.J,. Buring, J.E., Rosner, B., Hennekens, C.H., A prospective study of cigarette smoking and risk of cataract in men. Channing Laboratory, Department of Medicine, Harvard Medical School, Boston, MA. JAMA 1992 Aug 26;268(8):989-93.

Cohen-Addad C, Pares S, Sieker L, Neuburger M, Douce R., The lipoamide arm in the glycine decarboxylase complex is not freely swinging. Nat Struct Biol 1995 Jan;2(1):63-8.

Constantinescu, A., Pick, U., Handelman GJ, Haramaki N, Han D, Podda M. Tritschler HJ, Packer L Reduction and transport of α–Lipoic Acid by human erythrocytes. Biochem Pharmacol 1995 Jul 17;50(2):253-61.

Constantinescu, A., Tritschler, H., Packer, L., Alpha–Lipoic Acid protects against hemolysis of human erythrocytes induced by peroxyl radicals. The azo initiator of peroxyl radicals 2,2'-azobis Biochem Mol Biol Int 1994 Jul;33(4):669-79.

Culter, R.G., "Peroxide-producing potential of tissues: inverse coorelation with longevity of mammalian species" Pro Natl Acad. Sciences, 1985,82, pp 4,798-802.

Culter, R.G., "Carotenoids and retinol; their possible importance in determaning longevity of primate species.' Proc. Natl. Acad Science, 1984, 81, pp.7627-31.

Daniliak, I.G.; Kogan, A.K.; Bolevich, S., The generation of active forms of oxygen by the blood leukocytes, lipid peroxidation and antiperoxide protection in bronchial asthma patients. Ter Arkh 1992;64(3):54-7.

Deucher, G., Antioxidant therapy in the aging process. Clinica Guilherme Paulo Deucher, Sao Paulo, Brazil. EXS 1992;62:428-37.

Dimpfel, W., Spuler, M., Pierau, F.K 'Thioctic Acid Induces Dose-Dependent Sprouting of Neurites in Cultured Rat Neuroblastoma Cells" Developmental Pharmacology and Therapeutics 91990).14: 193-199.

Doelman, C.J., Bast, A., Oxygen radicals in lung pathology. Department of Pharmacochemistry, Faculty of Chemistry Vrije Universiteit, Amsterdam, The Netherlands. Free Radic Biol Med 1990;9(5):381-400.

Dorofeeva, G., Bondar, L., Lepikhov, P., Prilutskii, A., Characteristics of the functional state of the pancreas, lipid peroxidation and antioxidant defense in food hypersensitivity in children Pediatriia 1992;(3):18-22.

Faust, A.; Burkart, V.; Ulrich, H.; Weischer, C., Kolb, H. Effect of α–Lipoic Acid on cyclophosphamide-induced diabetes and insulitis in non-obese diabetic mice. Diabetes Research Institute, University of Dusseldorf, Germany. Int J Immunopharmacol 1994 Jan;16(1):61-6.

Flannery, G., Burroughs, A., Butler, P., Chelliah, J., Hamilton-Miller J., Brumfitt, W., Baum, H. Antimitochondrial antibodies in primary biliary cirrhosis recognize both specific peptides and shared epitopes of the M2 family of antigens. Hepatology 1989 Sep;10(3):370-4.

Freed, B., Rapoport. et. al., Inhibition of early events in the human T-lymphocyte response to mitogens and allogantigens by hydrogen peroxide. Arch Surg. (1987) 122: 99-104.

Fregeau, D., Roche, T., Davis, P., Coppel R., Gershwin M., J Immunol 1990 Mar 1;144(5):1671+.

Fujiwara, K., Okamura-Ikeda K, Motokawa Y., Lipoylation of H-protein of the glycine cleavage system. The effect of site-directed metagenesis of amino acid residues around the lipoyllysine residue on the lipoate attachment.

Fujiwara, K., Okamura-Ikeda, K., Motokawa, Y,. cDNA sequence, in vitro synthesis, and intramitochondrial lipoylation of H-protein of the glycine cleavage system. J Biol Chem 1990 Oct 15;265(29):17463-7.

Fujiwara. K., Okamura-Ikeda, K., Motokawa, Y. "Assay for protein lipoylation reaction." Institute for Enzyme Research, University of Tokushima, Japan. Methods Enzymol 1995;251:340-7.

Fussey, S., Bassendine, M., James, O., Yeaman, S., Characterisation of the reactivity of autoantibodies in primary biliary cirrhosis. Biochem Biophys Res Commun 1989 Jul 31;162(2):658-63.

Garganta CL, Wolf B , Lipoamidase activity in human serum is due to biotinidase. Clin Chim Acta 1990 Aug 31;189(3):313-25.

Gotz ME, Dirr A, Gsell W, Burger R, Janetzky B, Freyberger A, Reichmann H, Rausch WD, Riederer P Influence of N-methyl-4-phenyl-1,2,3,6-tetrahydropyridine, α–Lipoic Acid and L-deprenyl on the interplay between cellular redox systems. J Neural Transm Suppl 1994;43:145-62.

Gregus, Z., Stein, Varga, Effect of α–Lipoic Acid on biliary excretion of glutathione and metals. Toxicol Appl. Pharmcol (1992) 114: 86-96.

Gries, F.A., D. Ziegler, M. Hanefeld, K. J. Rulinau, H.B. MeiPner, "Symtomatic diabetic peripheral ItA4 neuropathy With the anti-oxidant alpha –Lipoic Acid: A 3-week multicentre randomized controlled trial" *Oxidants and Antioxidants in Biology*, Oxygen Club of California, Annual Meeting, March 1995.

Gut J, Christen U, Frey N, Koch V, Stoffler DMolecular mimicry in halothane hepatitis: biochemical and structural characterization of lipoylated autoantigens. Toxicology 1995 Mar 31;97(1-3):199-224.

Han, D. & Packer, L., "A-Lipoic Acid Modulation of Glutathione in a Human T-lymphocyte cell line." *Oxidants and Antioxidants in Biology*, Oxygen Club of California, Annual Meeting, March 1995

Han D, Handelman GJ, Packer LAnalysis of reduced and oxidized α–Lipoic Acid in biological samples by high-performance liquid chromatography. Methods Enzymol 1995;251:315-25.

Han D, Tritschler HJ, Packer L. Alpha–Lipoic Acid increases intracellular glutathione in a human T-lymphocyte Jurkat cell line. Biochem Biophys Res Commun 1995 Feb 6;207(1):258-64.

Haramaki, N., L, Packer et al "Cardiac Recovery During Post-Ischemic Reperfusion is Improved By Combination of Vitamin E With Dihydrolipoic Acid" Biochemical and Biophysical Research (1993). Vol 196, No. 3, 1101-1107.

Harding J.J., Cigarettes and cataract: cadmium or a lack of Vitamin C? [editorial; comment] Br J Ophthalmol 1995 Mar;79(3):199-200.

Hatch GE "Asthma, inhaled oxidants, and dietary antioxidants. Pulmonary Toxicology Branch, US Environmental Protection Agency, Research Triangle Park, NC Am J Clin Nutr 1995 Mar;61(3 Suppl):625S-630S.

Haugaard N., "Stimulation of Glucose Utilization By Thioctic Acid in Rat Diaphragm Incubated in vitro" Biochemica et Biophysica ACTA (1970). 583-586.

Heliovaara M; Knekt P; Aho K; Aaran RK; Alfthan G; Aromaa A Serum antioxidants and risk of rheumatoid arthritis. Social Insurance Institution, Helsinki, Finland. Ann Rheum Dis 1994 Jan;53(1):51-3.

Henrotin Y; Deby-Dupont G; Deby C; Franchimont P; Emerit I Active oxygen species, articular inflammation and cartilage damage. University Sart-Tilman. Liege, Belgium. EXS 1992 62:308-22.

Hofmann, M., Mainka, P., Tritschler, H., Fuchs, J., Decrease of red cell membrane fluidity and -SH groups due to hyperglycemic conditions is counteracted by α–Lipoic Acid. Arch Biochem Biophys 1995 Dec 1;324 (1): 85-92.

Honkanen., V., The factors affecting plasma glutathione peroxidase and selenium in rheumatoid arthritis: a multiple linear regression analysis. Scand J Rheumatol 1991;20(6):385-91.

Jacob, S., Henriksen, E., Schiemann A., Simon I, Clancy DE, Tritschler HJ. Jung WI "Enhancement of glucose disposal in patients with type 2 diabetes by α–Lipoic Acid." Arzneimittelforschung 1995 Aug;45(8):872-4.

Jayanthi, S.. Varalakshmi, P., Tissue lipids in experimental calcium oxalate lithiasis and the effect of DL α–Lipoic Acid. Department of Medical Biochemistry, Dr. A.L.M. P.G.I.B.M.S, University of Madras, India. Biochem Int 1992 Apr;26(5):913-21.

Jayanthi, S., Jayanthi, G., Varalakshmi, P., Effect of DL α–Lipoic Acid on some carbohydrate metabolizing enzymes in stone forming rats. Department of Medical Biochemistry, University of Madras, India Biochem Int 1991 Sep;25(1):123-36.

Jayanthi, S., Saravanan, N., Varalakshmi, P., "Effect of DL α–Lipoic Acid in glyoxylate-induced acute lithiasis." Department of Medical Biochemistry, Dr A.L. Mudaliar Post Graduate Institute of Basic Medical Sciences, University of Madras, India. Pharmacol Res 1994 Oct-Nov;30(3):281-8.

Jorg, J., Metz, F., Scharafinski, H., "Drug treatment of diabetic polyneuropathy with α–Lipoic Acid or Vitamin B preparations. A clinical and neurophysiologic study Neurologische Universitatskliniken Lubeck und Essen. Nervenarzt 1988 Jan;59(1):36-44.

Junqueira,V., Barros, A.P., Fuzaro, T., da Silva, S., Chan, V., et. al., "Decreasing Blood Oxidative Stress Status In Coronary Heart Disease Patients by Oral Antioxidant Supplementation" Oxidants and Antioxidants in Biology, Oxygen Club of California, Annual Meeting, March 1995.

Kagan, V., Freisleben, H., Tsuchiya, M., Forte, T., Packer, L., "Generation of probucol radicals and their reduction by ascorbate and dihydroα–Lipoic Acid in human low density lipoproteins. Department of Molecular and Cell Biology. University of California, Berkeley 94720. Free Radic Res Commun 1991; 15(5): 265-76.

Kagan, V., Shvedova, A., Serbinova, E., "Dihydrolipoic Acid - A Universal Antioxidant Both in the Membrane and in the Aqueous Phase. Reduction of Peroxyl, Ascorbyl and Chromanoxyl Radicals"

Kagan, V., Serbinova, E., Forte, T., Scita, G., Packer, L., "Recycling of Vitamin E in human low density lipoproteins." J Lipid Res 1992 Mar;33(3):385-97.

Kagan, V., Yalowich, J., Day, B., Goldman, R., Gantchev, T., Stoyanovsky, D.,

"Ascorbate is the primary reductant of the phenoxyl radical of etoposide in the presence of thiols both in cell homogenates and in model systems." Department of Environmental and Occupational Health, University of Pittsburgh, Pennsylvania 15238. Biochemistry 1994 Aug 16;33(32):9651-60.

Kahler W; Kuklinski B; Ruhlmann C; Plotz C [Diabetes mellitus--a free radical-associated disease. Results of adjuvant antioxidant supplementation] Klinik fur Innere Medizin, Klinikums Rostock-Sudstadt. Z Gesamte Inn Med 1993 May;48(5):223-32.

Kawabata T, Packer L, Alpha–lipoate can protect against glycation of serum albumin, but not low density lipoprotein. Biochem Biophys Res Commun 1994 Aug 30;203(1):99-104.

Kilic F., Packer. L., Trevethick, J.R. Modeling corticol cataracogenesis 17: Invitro effect of a α–Lipoic Acid on glucose-induced lens membrane damage, a model of diabetic cataractogenesis Exp. Eye Res (1994).

Kilic F; Handelman GJ; Serbinova E; Packer L; Trevithick JR Modelling cortical cataractogenesis 17: in vitro effect of α–α–Lipoic Acid on glucose-induced lens membrane damage, a model of diabetic cataractogenesis. Dept. of Biochemistry, University of Western Ontario, London, Canada. Biochem Mol Biol Int 1995 Oct;37(2):361-70.

Kis, K., Meier, T., Multhoff, G., Issels, R., Lipoate Modulation of Lymphocyte Cysteine Uptake, Institute for Klinische Hamatologie, GSF Forschungszentrum for Umwelt and Gesundeit.

Klein BE; Klein R; Linton KL; Franke T Cigarette smoking and lens opacities: the Beaver Dam Eye Study Department of Ophthalmology, University of Wisconsin, Madison. Am J Prev Med 1993 Jan-Feb;9(1):27-30, Comment in: Am J Prev Med 1993 Jan-Feb;9(1):65-6.

Komeshima N; Osawa T; Nishitoba T; Jinno Y; Kiriu T Synthesis and anti-inflammatory activity of antioxidants, 4-alkylthio-o-anisidine derivatives. Pharmaceutical Research Laboratory, Kirin Brewery Co., Ltd., Gunma, Japan. Chem Pharm Bull (Tokyo) 1992 Feb;40(2):351-6.

Korkina, L.G. Afanasef, I.B. et al Antioxidant therapy in children affected by irradiation from the Chernobyl nuclear accident. Biochem Soc. Trans (1993) 21: 314S.

Kropachova K., Mishurova E., Flavobion and thioctacid lessen irradiation-induced latent injury of the liver, Biull Eksp Biol Med 1992 May;113(5):547-9.

Lahoda F., Therapeutic possibilities in polyneuropathies Fortschr Med 1982 Oct 14;100(38):1759-60.

Legrand-Poels, S., Vaira D., et al. Activation of human immunodeficiency virus type 1 by oxidative stress. AIDS Res Human Retrovir (1990) 6: 1389-1397.

Leung PS, Iwayama T, Coppel RL, Gershwin MESite-directed metagenesis of lysine within the immunodominant autoepitope of PDC-E2. Division of Rheumatology, Allergy and Clinical Immunology, University of California,

Davis. Hepatology 1990 Dec;12(6):1321-8.

Lin, R.C., Antony, V., Lumeng L., Li, T.K., Mai, K., Liu, C., Wang, Q.D., et. al. Alcohol Clin Exp Res 1994 Dec;18(6):1443-7

Loffelhardt, S., Bonaventura, C., Locher, M., Borbe, H.O., Bisswanger, H., Interaction of alpha–Lipoic Acid enantiomers and homologues with the enzyme components of the mammalian pyruvate dehydrogenase complex. Biochem Pharmacol 1995 Aug 25;50(5):637-46

Low, P.A., K. Nickander, L.D. Schmelzer, M. Kihara, M. Nagamatsu & H. Tritschler "Experimental Diabetic Neuropathy: Idcremia, Oxidative Stress, and Neuroprotection" Mayo Fountaion and Asta Medica Dresdan, Germany *Oxidants and Antioxidants in Biology,* Oxygen Club of California, Annual Meeting, March 1995

Maitra, I., Serbinova, E., Trischler, H., Packer, L., Alpha–α–Lipoic Acid prevents buthionine sulfoximine-inducedcataract formation in newborn rats. Free Radic Biol Med 1995 Apr;18(4):823-9

Mares-Perlman, J.A.; Brady, W.E.; Klein, R.; Klein, B.E.; Bowen, P; Stacewicz-Sapuntzakis, M.; Palta, M. "Serum antioxidants and age-related macular degeneration in a population-based case-control study." Arch Ophthalmol 1995 Dec;113(12): 1518-23

Matsugo, S., Yan, L.J., Han, D., Trischler, H.J., Packer, L. Elucidation of antioxidant activity of alpha–α–Lipoic Acid toward hydroxyl radical. Biochem Biophys Res Commun 1995 Mar 8;208(1):161-7

McAlindon, T.E.; Jacques, P.; Zhang, Y.; et. al. Do antioxidant micronutrients protect against the development and progression of knee osteoarthritis? Arthritis Center,Boston U Med Cen, Arthritis Rheum 1996 Apr;39(4):648-56

McCarty, M.F.; Rubin, E.J., Rationales for micronutrient supplementation in diabetes. Med Hypotheses 1984 Feb;13(2):139-51

Mizuno, M., Packer, L., Suppression of protooncogene c-fos expression by antioxidant dihydroα–Lipoic Acid. Department of Molecular and Cell Biology, University of California, Berkeley. Methods Enzymol 1995;252:180-6

Morgan, M.Y., "Hepatoprotective agents in alcoholic liver disease. Acta Med Scand Suppl 1985;703:225-33

Morris, C.J.; Earl, J.R.; Trenam, C.W.; Blake, D.R., Reactive oxygen species and iron--a dangerous partnership in inflammation. Int J Biochem Cell Biol 1995 Feb;27(2):109-22

Muller, L. Menzel HTI - Studies on the efficacy of lipoate and dihydrolipoate in the alteration of cadmium2+ toxicity in isolated hepatocytes. Biochim Biophys Acta 1990 May 22;1052(3):386-91

Muller,. L. "Synergistic Effects of Alpha–Tocopherol and Alpha–Lipoic Acid on Reactive Oxygen Species in Blood" 57-64.

Nagamatsu. M, Nickander, K.K, Schmelzer, J.D., Raya, A., Wittrock, D.A.,

Tritschler, H., Low, P.A., "Lipoic Acid improves nerve blood flow, reduces oxidative stress, and improves distal nerve conduction in experimental diabetic neuropathy." Diabetes Care 1995 Aug;18(8):1160-7.

Nilsson, L., Ronge, E., Lipoamidase and biotinidase deficiency: evidence that lipoamidase and biotinidase are the same enzyme in human serum. Eur J Clin Chem Clin Biochem 1992 Mar;30(3):119-26.

Novak, Z.; Nemeth, I.; Gyurkovits, K,; Varga, S.I.; Matkovics B Examination of the role of oxygen free radicals in bronchial asthma in childhood. Clin Chim Acta 1991 Sep 30;201(3):247-51.

Olin, K.L.; Morse, L.S.; Murphy, C.; Paul-Murphy, J.; Line, S.; Bellhorn, R.W.; Hjelmeland, L.M.; Keen, C.L., Trace element status and free radical defense in elderly rhesus macaques (Macaca mulatta) with macular drusen. University of California, Davis 95616. Proc Soc Exp Biol Med 1995 Apr;208(4):370-7.

O'Neill, C.A., Halliwell, B., van der Vliet, A., Davis, P.A., Packer, L., Tritschler, H., Strohman, W.J., Rieland, T, Cross, C.E., Reznick, A.Z.. Aldehyde-induced protein modifications in human plasma: protection by glutathione and dihydroa-Lipoic Acid. J Lab Clin Med 1994 Sep;124(3):359-70.

Ou, P.; Tritschler, H.J.; Wolff, S.P., Thioctic (lipoic) acid: a therapeutic metal-chelating antioxidant? Department of Medicine, University College London Medical School, U.K. Biochem Pharmacol 1995 Jun 29;50(1):123-6.

Packer, L., "New horizons in Antioxidant Research: Action of Thioctic Acid/Dihydrolipic Acid Couple in Biological Systems" 35-45.

Packer, L., "Protective role of Vitamin E in biological systems. Department of Molecular and Cell Biology, University of California, Berkeley. Am J Clin Nutr 1991 Apr;53(4 Suppl):1050S-1055S.

Packer L., Suzuki, "Vitamin E and Alpha–Lipoate: Role in Antioxidant Recycling and Activation of the NF-KB Transcription Factor" Molec. Aspects med. (1993).

Packer, L., "New Horizons in 'Vitamin E Research - The Vitamin E Cycle, Biochemistry, and Clinical Applications" Lipid-Soluble Antioxidants: Biochemistry and Clinical Applications (1992).

Packer, L., Witt EH, Tritschler HJ "alpha–Lipoic Acid as a biological antioxidant." Free Radic Biol Med 1995 Aug;19(2):227-50.

Packer, L., Antioxidant properties of α–Lipoic Acid and its therapeutic effects in prevention of diabetes complications and cataracts. Ann N Y Acad Sci 1994 Nov 17;738:257-64.

Panigrahi, M., Sadguna, Y., et al "Alpha Lipid Acid Protects Against Reper-fusion Injury Following Cerebral lschemia in Rats" Brain Research (1996).

Parish, R.C., Doering P.L., Treatment of Amanita mushroom poisoning: a review Vet Hum Toxicol 1986 Aug;28(4):318-22.

Patel, M.S., Vettakkorumakankav NN, Liu TCDihydrolipoamide dehydrogenase: activity assays.Methods Enzymol 1995;252:186-95.

Paydas, S., Kocak, R., Erturk, F., Erken, E., Zaksu, HS., Gurcay, A.,Poisoning due to amatoxin-containing Lepiota species. Department of Internal Medicine, Cukurova University Medical School, Adana, Turkey. Br J Clin Pract 1990 Nov;44(11):450-3.

Pick, U., Haramaki, N., Constantinescu, A., Handelman, G.J, Tritschler HJ. Packer, L. Glutathione reductase and lipoamide dehydrogenase have opposite stereospecificities for α–Lipoic Acid enantiomers. Biochem Biophys Res Commun 1995 Jan 17;206(2):724-30.

Piering, W.F., Bratanow, N., Role of the clinical laboratory in guiding treatment of Amanitavirosa mushroom poisoning: report of two cases. Clin Chem 1990 Mar;36(3):571-4.

Podda, M., Tritschler, H.J., Ulrich, H., Packer, L. "α–Lipoic Acid supplementation prevents symptoms of Vitamin E deficiency." Department of Molecular and Cell Biology, University of California at Berkeley, 94720-3200. Biochem Biophys Res Commun 1994 Oct 14;204(1):98-104.

Podda, M., B. Koh, B. Descans, M. Rallis & L. Packer " Penetration, Reduction, and Protective Effects if α–Lipoic Acid in UV --Exposed Skin, Oxidants and Antioxidants in Biology, Oxygen Club of California, Annual Meeting, March 1995.

Powell, C.V.; Nash, A.A.; Powers, H.J.; Primhak, R.A. "Antioxidant status in asthma. Children's Hospital, Western Bank, Sheffield, United Kingdom. Pediatr Pulmonol 1994 Jul;18(1):34-8.

Ramakrishnan, Wolfe, Catravas. Radioprotection of hematopic tissues in mice by α–Lipoic Acid Radiation Research (1992) 130:360-365.

Ramakrishnan, S.; Sulochana, K.N.; Selvaraj, T.; Abdul Rahim A.; Lakshmi M.; Arunagiri, K., Smoking of beedies and cataract: cadmium and Vitamin C in the lens and blood Medical and Vision Research Foundations, Madras, India. Br J Ophthalmol 1995 Mar;79(3):202-6.

Ron, G.I.; Shmeleva, L.T.; Klein, A.V.; Iashkova, E., Lipid peroxidation and the status of the basal membrane of the acinar cells in the minor salivary glands of patients with Sjogren's syndrome. Stomatologiia (Mosk) 1992 Mar-Apr; (2):23-6.

Rosenberg, Hans, Culik, R., "Effect of DL Alpha Lipoic Acid in glyoxylate-induced Acute Lithiasis" The Italian Pharmacological Society (1994) Vol 80, 86-90.

Rucker, R.B., Wold, F., Cofactors in and as posttranslational protein modifications. FASEB J 1988 Apr;2(7):2252-61.

Sachse, G.; Willms, B. Efficacy of thioctic acid in the therapy of peripheral diabetic neuropathy. Horm Metab Res Suppl 1980; 9:105-7.

Said, H.M., Redha, R., Nylander, W.A. carrier-mediated, Na+ gradient-depen-

105

dent transport for biotin in human intestinal brush-border membrane vesicles.Vanderbilt University School of Medicine, Am J Physiol 1987 Nov; 253 (5 Pt 1):G631-6.

Scheer, B., Zimmer, G. DHLA prevents hypoxic/reoxygenation and peroxidative damage in rat heart mitochrondria. Arch Biochem Biophys. (1993) 302:385-390.

Schepkin, V., Kawabata. T., Packer L, "NMR study of α–Lipoic Acid binding to bovine serum albumin. Biochem Mol Biol Int 1994 Aug;33(5):879-86

Seaton, T.A., Jenner, P., "A Report on the Effects of Acute and Subacute Administration of R- and 5-Thioctic Acid on 14 C-Deoxyglucose Utilization in Rat Brain (1992).

Seddon, J.M.; Ajani, U.A.; Sperduto. R.D.; Hiller, R.; Blair, N.; Burton, T.C.; Farber, M.D.; Gragoudas, E.S.; Haller, J.; et al Dietary carotenoids, Vitamins A, C, and E, and advanced age-related macular degeneration. Eye Disease Case-Control Study Group [see comments] [published erratum appears in JAMA 1995 Feb 22;273(8):622] JAMA 1994 Nov 9;272(18):1413-20

Serbinova, E., Shamsuddin, K, et al, "Thioctic Acid Protects Against ischemiα–reperfusion injury In The isolated Perfused Langendorf Heart" Free Rad. Res. Comms (1992) Vol 17:1, 49-58

Shalini, V.K.; Luthra, M.; Srinivas, L.; Rao, S.H.; Basti, S.; Reddy, M.; Balasubramanian, D., Oxidative damage to the eye lens caused by cigarette smoke and fuel smoke condensates. Centre for Cellular and Molecular Biology, Hyderabad, India. Indian J Biochem Biophys 1994 Aug;31(4):261-6

Shvedova AA; Kisin ER; Kagan VE; Karol MH "Increased lipid peroxidation and decreased antioxidants in lungs of guinea pigs following an allergic pulmonary response. Toxicol Appl Pharmacol 1995 May;132(1):72-81

Shoji, S., Furuishi, K. Misumi, S., Miyazaki, T., Kino, M., Yamataka, K., Thiamine disulfide as a potent inhibitor of human immunodeficiency virus (type-1) production. Biochem Biophys Res Commun 1994 Nov 30;205(1):967-75

Smith, L.J.; Houston, M.; Anderson, J. Increased levels of glutathione in bronchoalveolar lavage fluid from patients with asthma. Am Rev Respir Dis 1993 Jun;147(6 Pt 1):1461-4

Snodderly, D.M. "Evidence for protection against age-related macular degeneration by carotenoids and antioxidant Vitamins." Schepens Eye Research Institute, Macular Disease Research Center, Am J Clin Nutr 1995 Dec;62(6 Suppl):1448S-1461S

Stoll, S., Hartmann, H., et al The potent rree radical scavanger α–Lipoic Acid improved memory in aged mice. Putative relationship to NMDA receptor deficits. Pharmacol. Biochem. Behav (1993) 36:799-805.

Strodter, D.; Lehmann, E.; Lehmann, U.; Tritschler, H.J.; Bretzel RG; Federlin K The influence of thioctic acid on metabolism and function of the diabetic heart. Medical Clinic III, University of Giessen, Germany. Diabetes

Res Clin Pract 1995 Jul;29(1):19-26

Studt,. J,; Heuer, L.J. Diabetic autonomic neuropathy of the heart and its treatment with thioctic acid Dtsch Z Verdau Stoffwechselkr 1984;44(4): 173-80

Sumathi, R,. Jayanthi, S. Kalpanadevi, V., Varalakshmi, P., "Effect of DL α–Lipoic Acid on tissue lipid peroxidation and antioxidant systems in normal and glycollate treated rats." Pharmacol Res 1993 May-Jun;27(4): 309-18.

Sumathi, R. Devi, and Varalakshmi, D., L α–Lipoic Acid protection against cadmiu,-induced tissue peroxidation Med Sci Res (1994) 22: 23-25.

Suzuki., Y.J., Mizuno, M., Tritschler, H.J., Packer, L., "Regulation of NF-kappa B DNA binding activity by dihydrolipoate.Department of Molecular & Cell Biology, Biochem Mol Biol Int 1995 Jun;36(2):241-6.

Suzuki YJ, Tsuchiya M, Packer L "Lipoate prevents glucose-induced protein modifications. Department of Molecular & Cell Biology, University of California, Berkeley 94720. Free Radic Res Commun 1992;17(3):211-217.

Suzuki YJ, Tsuchiya M, Packer L " Thiotic Acid and Dihydrolipoic Acid are Novel antioxidants which interact with reactive oxygen species" Free Rad. Res. Comm, (1991) Vol 15: 5 pp 255-263.

Spoerke, D.G., Smolinske, S.C., Wruk, K.M., Rumack, B.H Infrequently used antidotes: indications and availability. Vet Hum Toxicol 1986 Feb;28(1):69-75.

Teichert, J., Preiss, R.H., PLC-methods for determination of α–Lipoic Acid and its reduced form in human plasma.Institute of Clinical Pharmacology, University of Leipzig, Germany. Biochem Biophys Res Commun 1992 Dec 30; 189 (3):1709-15.

Teichert, J., Preiss, R. Determination of α–Lipoic Acid in human plasma by high-performance liquid chromatography with electrochemical detection. J Chromatogr B Biomed Appl 1995 Oct 20;672(2):277-81.

Trevino, R.J., "Air pollution and its effect on the upper respiratory tract and on allergic rhinosinusitis. Otolaryngol Head Neck Surg 1996 Feb;114(2): 239-41.

Trevithick, J.R., F. Kilic, G.J Handelman, E. Serbinow & L. Packer "In Vitro Effect of α–Lipoic Acid on Glucose-induced Lens membrane damage, a model of Diabetic Cataractgenesis" University of Western Ontario, London, Ontario, and University of California, Berkley, Oxidants and Antioxidants in Biology, Oxygen Club of California, Annual Meeting, March 1995.

Tritschler, P. HJ, Wolff, S.P., Thioctic (lipoic) acid: a therapeutic metal-chelating antioxidant? Biochem Pharmacol 1995 Jun 29;50(1):123-6.

Troisi, R.J.; Willett, W.C.; Weiss, S.T.; Trichopoulos, D.; Rosner, B.; Speizer F.E., A prospective study of diet and adult-onset asthma [see comments] Am J Respir Crit Care Med 1995 May;151(5):1401-8 Comment in: Am J Respir Crit Care Med 1995 May;151(5):1292-3.

Tsuchiya, Thompson, Suzuki, et. al., Superoxide fromed from cigarette smoke impairs polymorphononuclear leukocyte active oxygen generation activity. Arch Biochem Biophys (1992) 299: 30-37.

van der Vliet A, Cross CE, Halliwell B, O'Neill C., Plasma protein sulfhydryl oxidation: effect of low molecular weight thiols.department of Internal Medicine, UCD Medical Center, U of C, Sacramento Methods Enzymol 1995;251:448-55.

West, S.; Munoz, B.; Schein, O.D.; Vitale, S.; Maguire, M.; Taylor, H.R.; Bressler, N.M. Cigarette smoking and risk for progression of nuclear opacities. Dana Center for Preventive Opthalmology, Wilmer Institute, Johns Hopkins University, Baltimore, MD., Arch Ophthalmol 1995 Nov; 113(11):1377-80.

Whiteman, M., Tritschler, H., Halliwell, B. Protection against peroxynitrite-dependent tyrosine nitration and alpha 1-antiproteinase inactivation by oxidized and reduced α–Lipoic Acid.Neurodegenerative Disease Research Centre, King's College, London, UK. FEBS Lett 1996 Jan 22;379(1):74-6.

Wickramasinghe, S.N., Hasan, R.. In vitro effects of vitamin C, thioctic acid and dihydroa-Lipoic Acid on the cytotoxicity of post-ethanol serum. Department of Haematology, St Mary's Hospital Medical School, Imperial College of Science, London, U.K. Biochem Pharmacol 1992 Feb 4;43(3):407-11.

Yan, Liang-Jun & Lester Packer "A-Lipoic Acid Protects apoloproteins B-100 of Human Low Density liproteins against oxidative modifications mediated by Hypochlorite." *Oxidants and Antioxidants in Biology*, Oxygen Club of California, Annual Meeting, March 1995.

Yoshida, I., Sweetman, L., Kulovich, S., Nyhan, W.L., Robinson, B.H., Effect of α–Lipoic Acid in a patient with defective activity of pyruvate dehydrogenase, 2-oxoglutarate dehydrogenase, and branched-chain keto acid dehydrogenase. Kurume University, Japan. Pediatr Res 1990 Jan;27(1):75-9.

Yuichiro, J., Suzuki, Masahiki, "Thioctic Acid and Dihydrolipoic Acid Are novel Antioxidants Which Interact With Reactive Oxygen Species" Free Radical Research Comms. (1991) Vol 15:No. 5, 255-263.

Zhang, Hwang, Sevanian & Dwyer "Dependence of the LDL Oxidative Susceptibility on the LDL Cholesterolprotein Ratio and α–Tocopherol Content in Human Plasma" *Oxidants and Antioxidants in Biology*, Oxygen Club of California, Annual Meeting, March 1995.

Ziegler, D., Conrad, F., Ulrich, H. et. al., "Effects of Treatment with the Antioxidant Alpha Lipoic Acid on Cardiac Autonomic Neuropathy in NIDDM Patients - a 4-month Randomized Controlled Multicenter- Trial (DEKAN Study).

Index

AGEs 20-21

Age-related Macular Degeneration .65, 67

Aging ..7-9, 14, 16-17, 21, 35, 47, 71-72

AIDS .... .54, 75, 77

Alcoholism .... .28, 57, 88

Allergies 3, 6, 16, 28, 39-40, 90-96

Alzheimer's 8, 20

Antiglycation .... .21, 31

Antioxidant Defense System ...... .30, 66

Antioxidants .. 3, 6-11, 13, 16, 20-24, 26, 28, 30, 32, 34-36, 39-40, 42-45, 47, 57-58, 66-67, 69, 73, 75, 79-80, 85, 91, 93-94, 96-97

Arthritis 3, 6, 8, 11, 15-16, 19, 21, 28, 45-48, 57, 92, 95-96

Ascorbate 29-31, 66, 72-73, 75, 86

Asthma 3, 6, 8, 11, 16, 28, 40-44, 96

ATP 6, 25, 50, 56, 82, 94

Blood 11, 15, 17, 20-22, 27, 31, 37-44, 47-55, 59-60, 67-68, 70-71, 73, 79-82, 89, 96

Blood Sugar 11, 20-22, 31, 49-52, 89

C-deficiency .... .24

Cadmium Toxicity .... .71, 86

Cancer 3, 6, 8, 13-18, 21, 33, 35-36

Capillary .... .14, 17

Carcinogens .... .15, 33

Cardiovascular Disease ...... .13, 17, 66

Carotenoids ...... .22, 26-27, 65, 67-69

Cataracts 3-4, 6, 8, 14,16-17, 49, 51-52, 65, 69-73

Cadmium toxicity .... .25, 86

Cholesterol .... .84

Cigarettes 4,10, 65, 69-70, 85

Collagen 14-15, 17, 20-21, 36

Cross-linking 8

Cysteine ..... .22, 27-28, 52, 77, 88, 95

Diabetes ..3, 6, 8, 11, 13, 16, 21, 28, 32, 49-54, 57-58-60, 66, 69, 71-74, 83-84, 89--96

Diabetic Peripheral Neuropathy 61-62

Diabetic Retinopathy 66, 71

Dihydrolipoic Acid 24-25, 66

Dosage 32, 59-60, 89-92, 96

Drusen 65, 67-68

E-deficiency 24

Energy 6, 10, 56, 94

Exercise 11, 56, 64

Eye 3, 16, 65, 68, 71

Foam cells 18-19

Free Radical Diseases 3, 13

Free Radicals 3, 6-10, 13-21, 23-24, 26-27, 30-31, 33-36, 39-45, 47, 52, 57, 64, 70, 72, 81-82, 85, 96

GABA 27

Genetic 8, 14-15, 33-35, 75

Glucose 20, 25, 27, 49-56, 59, 66, 72-74, 89-91, 94

Glutamic 27, 44

Glutathione .22, 26-32, 36-37, 41, 44, 46, 52, 58-61, 69, 72-73, 75, 77-79, 86, 88, 91, 95, 97

Glycation ...20-21, 31, 49, 52- 54, 81, 83

H2O2 . . . . .25, 46, 48, 86

Heart Disease . 3, 6, 8, 13-16, 18-19, 21, 49, 79

Heart Attack .81

Heavy Metals 6, 20, 25, 85

Hemoglobin 14, 41, 81

HIV 75-76, 78, 95

HOCl 25, 80-81

HPAL 61-62

Hydroperoxy 10, 32

Hydroxy 25

Hypochlorous 24-25, 80

Inflammation 3, 39, 46, 95

Insulin 21, 49-53, 66

Iron 9-10, 31, 46, 81

Irradiation 10, 35-37

Ketone bodies 54, 84

Kidney Stones 84

Lens 70-74

Lipid . 8, 19, 30-31, 35, 40, 42-43, 48, 67, 75, 80, 82, 84-86

Lipid Peroxidation 80

Lipoate 53-54, 64, 66, 72-73, 76, 84, 86, 95

Lipoic Acid Recycles 26

Lipoprotein 14, 18, 28, 79

Liver 6, 17, 30, 32, 36-37, 52, 54, 80, 83, 86-88, 97

Lupus .57, 92

Lycopene .68

Lysosomal .8

Macrophages 18-19, 39-40, 42

Macular Degeneration . . . 3, 6, 16, 49, 65, 67-69

Membrane . .7-8, 14, 17, 27-30, 34-35, 52, 59, 86

Memory .62-63

Metabolic Acidosis 54

Metal-Chelating Antioxidant 85

Mitochondria 14, 57, 63

Muscles 51-52, 56, 63

Mushroom Poisoning 87-88

N-acetylcysteine 77-78

N-methyl-o-aspartate 63

NADH 50

Nerve 16, 20, 49, 51-52, 55, 57-61
   Lipoic Acid Reverses Nerve Damage .58

Neurological Damage 20

Neuropathy . . .6, 52, 55, 57-62, 88-89, 91

NF-kappa B 34, 75-77, 95

NIDDM 53

Nitrogen 10, 42

NO2 10

Non-insulin dependent diabetes 50

O2 .25, 46, 71

O3 10

OH .10, 19, 45

Osteoarthritis 19, 45-47

Oxidants 9-10, 16-17, 26, 39, 42, 85

Oxidation . . .13, 14-17, 19, 23, 25-28, 30, 35, 45, 49, 52, 55, 57-58, 60-65, 67, 71- 73, 75-76, 78-81, 83-85, 95

Oxygen 8-10, 16-22, 24-25, 28, 34-35, 41, 43, 45-47, 57, 59, 71, 80-81

Oxygen Free Radicals 9-10, 45

Ozone 10

Packer . 16, 23, 27, 29-30, 36, 45, 51, 66, 73, 76, 78, 80-82, 87-88, 90, 93-97

Pain 15, 45, 47, 52, 59, 61

Parkinson's 20, 64

Peroxinorm 19, 45

Peroxyl 24-25, 30-32

Plaque 15, 18-19

Platelets 40, 42-43

Polyneuropathy 55

Polyunsaturated 14

PPP 42

Protein . . 7-8, 10,14, 16-18, 20-21, 26, 31, 34, 53-54, 71- 73, 77, 80-81, 83, 85, 94

Psoriasis 47-48

R-a-Lipoic Acid 74

Radiation 6, 10-11, 15, 33, 36-37, 69

Regenerates Nerves 55

Reperfusion 41, 59, 81-82

Retinopathy 16, 49, 52, 58, 66, 71

S-a-Lipoic Acid 74

SDN 59-61

Serbinova 29, 80, 82
Side Effects 32, 52, 90, 92, 96

Singlet oxygen 24-25, 71

Sjogren's Syndrome 48

Skin13, 15, 20, 30, 34-36, 46-47, 52, 80, 90, 96

Smoking 4,10, 65, 69-70, 85

SOD 22

Stress .. 11, 17, 27, 52, 55, 57, 60-61, 73, 75-76, 78-79, 83, 95

Stroke 81-82

Sugar 11, 20-22, 27, 31, 49-52, 83, 89

Superoxide . 10, 22, 24-26, 30, 32, 45, 58, 71, 79-80

Suzuki 54, 76-77

T-lymphocytes 75, 77

Thiols 40, 66, 73, 77, 86

Tocopherols 68

Topical ALA 35

Triglyceride 84

Type I Diabetes 50

Type II Diabetes 50-51, 53, 61

UV Radiation .11, 13, 15, 35-36, 69, 72, 96

Viruses 6, 9, 57, 75-76, 95

Vitamin B-1 .... 57, 94

Vitamin B-2 94

Vitamin C .. .22-24, 29-30, 42, 47, 66-67, 69-71, 73-74, 91, 96-97

Vitamin E .. 11, 22-24, 26-32, 36-37, 40-41, 44, 47, 58-59, 65-73, 79-80, 82, 89, 91, 96-97

Water Soluble 6, 31, 35, 71, 91

Wrinkles 15, 17

BOOKS AVAILABLE FROM BL PUBLICATIONS:

Health Learning Handbooks

Castor Oil: Its Healing Properties
by Beth Ley   36 pages, $3.95

Dr. John Willard on Catalyst Altered Water
By Beth Ley 60 pages, $3.95

How to Fight Osteoporosis and Win! The Miracle of Microcrystalline Hydroxyapatite
By Beth Ley   80 pages, $6.95 *

The Potato Antioxidant: Alpha Lipoic Acid
By Beth Ley   112 pages, $6.95 *

Additional Titles

Natural Healing Handbook
by Beth Ley with foreword by Dr. Arnold J. Susser,
R.P., Ph.D. 320 pages, $14.95 *

How Did We Get So Fat? *
By Dr. Arnold J. Susser and Beth Ley, 96 pages,
$7.95

A Diet For The Mind By Fred Chapur, 112 pages,
$8.95

DHEA: Unlocking the Secrets of the Fountain of Youth by Beth Ley, 208 pages, $14.95 *

* *Order by calling toll free:* ***1-800-507-2665***

You may also send book order total amount plus $2
shipping by check or money order to:
BL Publications, 21 Donatello, Aliso Viejo, CA 92656